Drops of Reality 4

More tales from a doctor's surgery ... and beyond

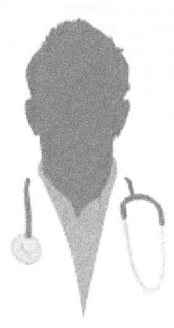

By Dr M. A. Moss

Drops of Reality 4
Independently published, 2024.
Copyright © Dr M.A. Moss, 2024.
ISBN: 9798332467660.

Formatting and cover design: Jim Bruce,
www.ebooklover.co.uk

Praise for the 'Drops of Reality' series

There are books on my shelves that I never loan out. I return to these books many times over the years to re-read and savour. "Drops of Reality" has been placed on my Kindle shelves as a favoured book. Dr Moss's stories are familiar to me because I was married to an NHS doctor for 26 years and I hear the ring of truth. It's a very enjoyable book and I sincerely hope Dr Moss writes another.

– Dorothy Franklin, American reviewer on Amazon

A very enjoyable book. It showed the humanity in a GP profession, which we generally don't get to see as they are so busy. Some tales were thought-provoking while others made me giggle out loud! I enjoyed the human element to the book and would recommend it in an instant.

– Debi, Amazon reviewer

Well told, funny and sad, showing the frailties and strengths of people in general. Would think such a caring doctor would be a blessing to any health service.

– Nicky, Amazon reviewer

I find that the series just keeps on getting better and better I can't wait for the next book.

– Lydia, Amazon reviewer

Fifteen short stories that make you laugh and cry, and sometimes teach you unexpected things about life, health and happiness. I only wish it had been longer....Can't wait for a sequel....

– Amazon reviewer

Contents

Introduction

First, I would like to thank my wonderful readers for their continued encouragement, and the positive feedback received for the previous three books in this series. Your support has provided me with much of the motivation to write another one. This time I have explored, in more depth, the stories of some of my patients, alongside subjects such as personal observations and life experiences.

I would also like to thank my friends, family and the writers' club for their continued help and advice; my staff and patients for the inspiration they have given me; and I would like to extend a special thanks to my colleague, Dr Clyde Saldanha, and my very helpful editor and formatter, Jim Bruce, of ebooklover.co.uk.

Although the stories in this book are very much true, I have changed the names and some identifiable details for the sake of confidentiality.

I hope you enjoy reading these stories as much as I enjoyed writing them.

Dr M A Moss, London, 2024

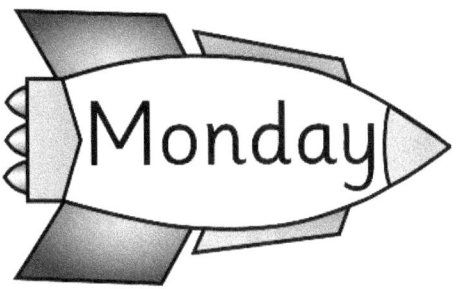

Chapter One
Another Manic Monday

The day began with a cloudless, blue sky, and the sunshine filled me with positive energy at the start of my working week as I left the house to drive to the surgery.

Traffic was heavy in the morning rush-hour and the school run, and at a small roundabout at the top of our street one hasty motorist had hit the bumper of another vehicle and the two drivers had pulled over to the side of the road to swap insurance details. I switched on the car radio to hear of major hold-ups on the M25 motorway.

Approaching the clinic, I stopped at a red traffic light at a crossroads. A woman driver across the way was looking at me and shouting, while waving her hands around. I tried to figure out what I'd done wrong, but then realised she was arguing with someone else on a hands-free phone.

The weather suddenly changed for the worse, with grey clouds dominating the sky and rain drizzling on my windscreen.

Arriving at the clinic, I parked my car and noticed an ambulance in the car park. Its crew, in their distinctive green uniforms, were taking one of my patients, Mrs Gonzales, to the local hospital.

She saw me, nodded in acknowledgement and waved her hand. I greeted her with a smile.

"Good morning, Mrs Gonzales, you will be fine and in safe hands at the hospital," I said.

I noticed vapour coming out of her oxygen mask, as if she was smoking or vaping. I remember that I told her, on her last appointment that if she needed help to quit smoking our nurses would be happy to help. But she was adamant she wanted to continue smoking.

I recall her saying, "It's an addiction, doctor. You know that". Her daughter Maria was with her at that consultation, where a heated debate erupted between the two of them. Maria told her mum, "You have to stop smoking" and Mrs Gonzales answered, "That's rich, coming from you. Can you stop drinking alcohol?"

One of the ambulance crew approached me, saying, "Good morning, Doc. Mrs Gonzales has had a severe asthma attack. Alisha, the nurse, and Dr Dikko tried to help, but it was decided that she needs to go to the local hospital for further tests, observation and treatment."

"Good luck, guys," I said, and I rushed into the clinic to avoid running late for my patient consultations.

The reception area was already almost full, with many familiar faces, and I said "Good morning, everybody." But my greetings were rudely interrupted by a screaming baby, whom I assumed had just had a vaccination. Then another two babies, who looked like twins, in a single pram, joined in the cacophony, probably in sympathy or solidarity with the other baby. Maybe they guessed the vaccination needle was also coming their way.

I tried to pass reception with a smile and greetings, but the response was, "Sorry, doctor, to jump on you first thing in the morning, but Mr Self ran out of his medications when he was away. He rang us many times for it, but you know him, he likes to complain. It's on your desk if you can sign it, please."

I nodded and headed straight to my room to start the morning session before some other problem arose.

I switched on my computer, which was slow to start, and I had to go through the usual many layers of secure access, with numerous passwords to remember.

I glanced at Mr Self's prescription before signing it, and I noticed that one item in his medications had been printed twice, so I printed it again with the correct items, to avoid him complaining.

Looking at my patient list, and some screen messages, I recognised many names, and I decided to start the session.

I called in the first patient, Rebecca, a single mum in her mid-twenties. I noted that the reason for her appointment was that her house had been burgled; she was distressed and needed help.

"Hello, Rebecca, how can I help?"

With a sad face, she said in a faint voice, "Good morning, doctor", paused for a few seconds, then grabbed a tissue from the tissue box on my desk, and started crying.

"I need a letter to the council to give me a flat with a secured entrance and with better ventilation, as the mould is filling the bathroom and the bedrooms, affecting our health, especially Ellie with her asthma.

"You remember what happened to me in my flat, and you sent me for counselling, when two hooded burglars knocked on my door and when I opened it, they pushed me aside with my kid. One of the burglars was wearing a long leather glove and he held my dog by the collar around her neck and she was frightened. The other intruder got hold of the two puppies, and they sped off in a car waiting outside in the street. I heard later from people that they sell the dogs for cash, as the cost of living is affecting many people.

"I couldn't stay in the flat, so I went to my mother's two-bedroom flat and stayed there. That put more stress on her and made her depression worse, adding to her recent anxiety of some teenage hooligans on the rough estate vandalising her car, thinking it was fun. These hooligans are known on the estate and the police are aware of their graffiti on the doors of local shops, and other antisocial behaviour, and cautioned them.

"Ellie, my seven-year-old daughter, after we sorted the bullying issues at her school, you know she is allergic to almost everything in life, except the dogs, as she grow up with them. However, she is clearly allergic to my mum's cat, with tense skin itchiness, red eyes, and continuous sneezing. So my mum had to ask her neighbour to have the cat for a few days, now it's been a few weeks, and Mum is missing her cat dearly.

"Despite us cleaning the room and Mum's house of all the cat fur, Ellie is still itching day and night, adding to her crying in the middle of the night with flashbacks of what she had seen of the burglars."

Rebecca paused to draw breath, then added, "And by the way, Doc, I received a letter from the allergy clinic. Thank you, Doc, for the referral, but they wanted me to take with us anything Ellie is allergic to. I can't take half of the supermarket food products, and I certainly can't take the cat with us!"

I tried to calm Rebecca and explain the routine letter which the hospital sends to everybody. I typed up a supporting letter to the council outlining her circumstances, requesting urgent help with her issues, and booked her again with the counselling service for support in her ordeal. I got a satisfied smile, at least for now.

(Almost a year later, I learned that Rebecca had been given better, more secured accommodation, with no mould, and she was very happy. Ellie's condition improved with treatment, and the dog had another two puppies to keep the family amused. Rebecca learned how to sell them on the internet, to a nice household to look after them, and got some extra money.)

* * * * *

My next patient was Paul, a young and fit police officer. Everybody in his family was proud of him, and he usually had a very positive attitude towards life. I'd known him from his teenage years, but this time he looked as if he'd been beaten-up by somebody.

"Good morning, young man. How are you?" I said.

Paul replied softly, "Not good, I'm afraid, Doc. I was attending a nasty domestic violence incident yesterday, where the drunk and very violent partner turned against us. I was trying to hold him away from his partner when he was attacking her. I got a hit in my leg, face and arm. Thankfully the situation was settled, we took him to the station and sorted him out."

I checked Paul over, and there were extensive bruises on his thigh, a small one near his cheek, and his arm, but luckily no bone fractures. I prescribed pain relief and gave him a sick note for a week to recover, telling him to report back to us if he needed more time off work.

Paul replied, "I don't think I'll need more than a week. I was even thinking of asking you that if I feel OK after three or four days, could I go back to work, as we are short-staffed?"

I was impressed by his dedication to duty, and with a smile said, "Yes you can". I offered him counselling for his psychological trauma but he mentioned that the force supplied that help for affected staff.

As Paul left the room, I thought about rising violence against police, hospital staff and ambulance crews. It made me wonder: what's gone wrong with our society?

* * * * *

After a few seconds of reflection, it was time for my next patient, with shoulder pain, as logged on the computer.

Mr Rana entered with another young man, a distant relative, to translate for him. His name was Mr Gurung, and both of them were in their early 40s, wearing neat casual clothes.

I noticed from the records that Mr Rana, originally from Nepal, was a relatively new patient to our clinic. He'd had a few previous consultations with our Dr Newman, who had sent him for an X-ray on his shoulder after he slipped on a wet floor at the food factory where he worked.

I checked the X-ray and he had no fracture. He had seen the nurses for blood tests and blood pressure monitoring, as his readings were high. He'd also had an ultrasound of the kidneys, as he had the occasional dull ache in the left loin, and discomfort with a scar on his right loin.

I concentrated on his shoulder problem, examining his painful and stiff shoulder. I agreed with Dr Newman about a diagnosis of frozen shoulder. She'd prescribed him strong pain relief, and physiotherapy exercises, but it hadn't helped much, and the poor man couldn't work with his pain, which meant no money for his family back in Nepal.

With Mr Gurung translating, I told Mr Rana I'd give him a steroid injection in his shoulder. While I was preparing the injection, Mr Gurung asked me about Mr Rana's blood tests, and I reassured him that it was all fine. Then he asked about the ultrasound results and I explained that it showed one absent kidney and a good other kidney, with no serious disease.

Silence filled the room for a few seconds, then I was asked a specific question about the right-side kidney: Had it start to grow?

I looked at the ultrasound again, which showed there was no right-side kidney, as I'd mentioned to them just minutes earlier.

"Yes, it has been removed, but that was five years ago. Surely it must have started to grow again?"

Baffled, I asked Mr Gurung what on earth he was talking about, while I checked Mr Rana's right loin, which showed a scar from the presumed kidney operation.

Mr Gurung said, "Mr Rana comes from a village called Hokse, east of the capital Kathmandu, nicknamed 'the kidney village'. Almost every house in the village has somebody who sold their kidney for money. They are poor, desperate for money, and they are approached by organ-trafficking middlemen, convincing them to sell one of their kidneys, explaining that doctors said we can live with only one kidney. Not only that, as time goes by the removed kidney will grow again, but it takes time.

"The deal was for around two thousand pounds. The person who agrees to sell their kidney will be taken to India, where the operation takes place. After a few days of recovery, they are handed the money and they return to their families, to feed them with the money gained. It's a very common practice in that village.

"Then some of these men, like Mr Rana, can be offered to be smuggled to England to work like a slave for a little more money, but it is more than enough for their families in Nepal to live on."

I listened in disbelief about this bizarre situation, and that it could be happening in the 21st century. But who was I to judge or change the world? I thought. I had better treat him to get him back to work and sending his earnings to his family in Nepal.

I explained, gently, that when a kidney is removed, it doesn't grow again, but that our bodies are designed so that they can function with just one kidney.

I was glad that Mr Rana's facial expression showed him starting to relax, giving me the impression that he'd accepted these facts, and had probably decided to live happily with just one kidney.

The consultation ended with big smiles from both of them – a common international language which needed no translation.

* * * * *

An administration note popped up on my computer screen, saying that a new patient, Duncan James, who had gone to the branch surgery and intimidated the staff, was requesting an urgent sick note for the Job Centre, as he had no money to buy food.

The duty doctor at the branch surgery had gone off for home visits, so I decided to help. I reckoned it should only take me about five minutes, and then I'd be ready to see more patients.

But I was wrong, as it took five minutes alone to go through his medical record of extensive physical, psychological, social and forensic history. It listed things like a motorcycle accident 10 years ago, an assault with a broken nose and facial bones, anxiety, depression, emotionally unstable personality, alcohol and drug misuse, Forensic history of shoplifting and hitting a Policeman.

He was on multiple medications, so I decided to ring him, to check his well-being and his current illness, before I wrote out a sick note. I noticed he had two numbers on his medical record: a landline and a mobile.

I chose the landline, as mobile reception is sometimes not good.

I dialled the number and put the call on speaker phone. While waiting for a response, I glanced at his medical record for more information, and was absorbed by the plethora of problems.

The call was suddenly answered, with a gentle female voice saying something quickly, which I missed, then "Can I help?"

I swiftly picked up the phone. "Good day, may I please talk to Mr Duncan James."

The woman replied, "No, you can't. Can I help you in any way?"

"I'm his doctor and he asked for help. Never mind, I'll try to get him on his mobile number."

The lady's voice became very authoritarian. "We don't allow mobile phones, according to the prison protocol."

I realised that the landline was not his home number, but the prison number. I thanked the lady, and called Mr James on his mobile.

He answered in a harsh voice, "Who is this?"

I introduced myself, and asked him how I could help him. He started telling me about his recent release from jail, the right wrist pain from the tight handcuffs applied by the police and the prison staff when he had been detained for something he claimed was trivial.

He said he'd asked a corner shop to give him a packet of cigarette and he would pay later when he got some money.

"The shop owner refused, so I had to show him a pair of scissors I was carrying for my personal use. He gave me a box of cigarettes, but I forgot there were CCTV cameras. He reported the incident to the police, who recognised me and came to arrest me.

"I'm going to sue them, and even their boss, that tough cookie, nice-looking Home Secretary, for my wrist problem. It's a human rights issue, Doc, but I can't write out a complaint because my wrist is hurting."

I decided I had enough information and I issued him with a sick note to collect and give to the Job Centre, and to book a future appointment for further investigations of his wrist pain, and a medication review. I gave him pain relief, a blood test and offered smoking-cessation help.

So much for a quick, five-minute administration job, I thought.

* * * * *

My next patient was Sanjita, a young, attractive Indian lady in her mid-thirties, tall and slim, with long, silky jet-black hair and wide brown eyes. She worked as an administrator for a charity organisation.

She had hit her elbow on the dining table two days earlier, and she also wanted to discuss her IBS (Irritable Bowel Syndrome).

After checking her elbow, I reassured her there was no bone fracture and it was only soft tissue swelling, which should subside in a few days with simple pain relief.

Moving on to her irritable bowel problem, she told me she had been following all the advice given by the specialist and the dietician, but the condition had repeatedly flared up.

I pointed out that there must be a cause, something like stress. I think she was waiting for me to say that word, as her facial expression revealed a sadness she was trying hard to conceal.

Sanjita explained the stressful situation at her work, with targets and deadlines, but the major issue was her heavy-drinking husband, Raj. After his hard working day as a builder, he kept arguing with her over trivial things, kept starting trouble between her and her daughter, Sonia, and wouldn't play a role model as a stepdad when she got married to him after a messy divorce from her ex-husband.

She told me how she had supported Raj until he got his permanent residency and British citizenship and got him a job. All she got in return were bad moods, arguments and abuse. Despite many attempts by Sanjita, and our clinic team, to convince him to get help for his drinking problem, he refused on many occasions.

One of the options was to refer her to a family counselling service, which could take weeks due to pressure on the system. Alternatively, I mentioned that if she had trustworthy close friends or relatives, they could act as counsellors. Sanjita dismissed these options, so the last recourse was the local religious temple, but her response was even more negative.

"They are good at taking donations and charity, but offer little or no help, even gossiping about things," she said.

This statement didn't surprise me as I'd heard similar accounts from some other patients, with different faiths, over many years.

We settled for extra medications to help Sanjita's IBS, I referred her for family counselling, and wished her good luck.

I decided to have a glass of water before I dealt with the next patient. Returning to my room, I could hear the phone ringing on my desk. Reception said the coroner's office was on the line, asking about one of our patients, who had passed away in the local hospital's intensive care unit in the early hours of this morning.

The coroner's officer introduced herself and told me that the poor young man, aged 31, had been found collapsed in the toilet in his shared accommodation by his flat mate. An ambulance crew, who took him to hospital, found many empty boxes of paracetamol in his room. He was resuscitated in hospital and admitted to the intensive care unit, as he'd suffered multi-system failures of his liver, kidneys and heart. Sadly, he had passed away.

As I listened to this story I looked at his medical record, which didn't show much, as he was a new patient, registered about six months ago after he joined a school studying business. He never came for any health check, despite many invitations from the clinic.

The coroner's officer asked me, "Did he get any paracetamol from your surgery at any time, and for what reason?"

I replied, "No, and he was not on any medication."

The officer requested a summary for their records and for the inquest, which I promised to draft at the end of my clinical work and email it to them.

* * * * *

A message flashed up on my computer screen: "When you have a minute, please ring our patient, Abimbola, regarding her weight management referral, as it had been rejected."

I had a few minutes to spare, so I rang her.

"Hello, Abimbola, how can I help?"

"Doc, I'm eating like a horse."

"That's why I referred you to the weight management team."

"I've tried to put on weight, but I can't!"

That sentence confused me, as I thought she was doing her best to lose weight. So why was she eating like a horse then?

I repeated, "That's why we referred you to weight management, to help you, and that is good."

"No, Doc, it's not good, because I received a letter from weight management saying I don't fit the criteria, as my weight is 117kg and it should be 119kg to make my BMI (Body Mass Index) of 40, then I would fit the criteria."

"Ah, I've got it. OK, Abimbola, leave it with me," I replied.

I delegated the issue to the hard-working Veronica, asking her to ring weight management on my behalf, and get them to waive the criteria this time, as Amibiola couldn't eat any more. She was desperate as she was getting married in three months and wanted to impress her partner.

I calmed Abimbola, and reassured her that our team would do their utmost to help her.

Later that day, a message popped up on my screen from Veronica, to let me know that weight management had waived the criteria for Amibiola, and had accepted her to start the programme soon. That was comforting news, and it made me happy.

* * * * *

My next patient was Mr Dogo. That's not his surname, but his nickname, which he preferred me to call him. He had explained it to me one day, saying he was the youngest of his brothers and sisters, and his granddad had twenty eight grandsons and granddaughters, and he found it difficult to remember all their names in his old age. So he decided to call him Dogo, which meant 'the little one' in their tribal language.

Mr Dogo recently had his blood test results, and the duty doctor noticed that his blood sugar level was getting higher, despite being on multiple oral medications for that. He had been invited in today for a review with me.

Mr Dogo was in his late fifties, tall, well built, of African origin, with a family history of diabetes. A family man, he worked hard as a taxi driver.

I recalled his last consultation with me, when he complained about Erectile Dysfunction ED (weak erection). As he described it, it was not like when he was thirty years old. ED is common among people who have had diabetes for a long time, with an uncontrolled sugar level.

We had supplied him with the well-known blue tablets, which worked initially. But then it was back to square one, so we changed it to the white tablet, and another one, and eventually we referred him to the hospital team for further management. The hospital wrote back to say they'd given him a pump to try, and taught him about the local injection in his private parts before intercourse.

I had repeatedly advised him to stick to the diabetic diet, and to take his medications regularly.

I called him in, and with his usual cheery disposition and friendly smile he said, "Good morning, my doctor."

"Good morning, Mr Dogo. How are you?" I replied.

"I'm fine, Doc. They asked me to see you."

I looked at the computer screen message about his high sugar level, and I explained it and the implications of it. His oral medications for diabetes were at the maximum strength, so he might need to go on insulin injections to control his diabetes better. If so, it would require him to do regular daily checks of his blood sugar level before he drove his taxi, and to have a good diabetic control otherwise it would be difficult to renew his cabbie's licence.

He interrupted me gently with a shy gaze, looking down at the floor, and apologised that he'd lost control when he was indulging in sweets, cakes and chocolates at recent family celebrations for birthdays and wedding anniversaries.

He also said he'd missed his diabetes medication sometimes, as well as his blood pressure medication. I noticed the last reading of his blood pressure was high.

When I tried to explain this point, he told me, "Doc, you advised me to buy a blood pressure machine, which I did, and when I'm relaxed at home, with the wife at work and no arguments, no bad news on the television, and no surprising bills, the reading is fine".

He then added "You told me before to try to avoid stress. But last week I was doing a night shift, when three drunk guys hailed my cab. On the way, they asked me to stop and wait while they bought fish and chips, and then they started eating it in the back of the car.

"When I told them that they could wait till they got home, they just kept eating, and laughing. When we arrived at their destination, they got out, saying they would get the money from inside the house.

"I waited for a long time, and when I rang the doorbell a different man answered and told me off. I thought, what's the point in shouting and making a scene, or even contacting the police? It would be my word against theirs, with no evidence like a mobile phone text for the taxi booking, or a CCTV recording. And the police must be very busy with other priorities, God help them."

Mr Dogo then suddenly reached down and took off his shoes and socks, showing me his discoloured toenails, and the peeling skin between his toes.

It was a fungal nail infection – a common complaint with people with diabetes, which reduces their immunity and makes an infection like this more commonplace.

I took a sample from a nail for laboratory analysis and gave him treatment, advising him to avoid getting warm and sweaty feet, and to wear cotton socks and leather shoes.

I thought he'd got the message, and with a wide smile he changed the subject to the good news about his last hospital review for his erectile dysfunction issue. The injection in his private part was working well.

Before I concluded the consultation, his face showed concern as he told me, "Now that the erectile dysfunction had been sorted, we celebrated the 50th birthday of my wife. I didn't realise that my wife, who was very demanding in the past, had gone into her menopause, with no desire for intimate relations, with many excuses. Can you help her, Doc?"

"Mr Dogo, you know we can't discuss your wife's health because of confidentiality. Please let her book an appointment to see our lady doctor, and I'm sure she will try to help sort this problem out for her," I reassured him.

I was about to say "Have a nice day" when he pulled out forms from a plastic folder he was carrying and said, "My daughter, you know her, she is applying for a midwifery course, and they wanted these forms from her doctor."

"That's fine, I'll do it for her, and I'll leave it in reception for her to collect. Have a good day, Mr Dogo."

* * * * *

Another message flashed up on the screen: "Mrs Muradi, upset, crying, wants to talk to you."

I thought it was probably the anniversary of her late husband's death, or that she was in pain from her arthritis, so I rang her between seeing two patients.

"Hello, Mrs Muradi, how can I help?"

"Doctor, I'm not well. I didn't sleep at all last night, as my two daughters and their husbands came to visit me over the weekend, and they were talking about the boss of my younger daughter, his name is Mr Kazemi, who attended her wedding and saw me at the wedding, where he had a long chat with me. He is divorced and a very wealthy British businessman of Iranian origin, who has settled in the UK for decades. He wanted to propose to me.

"I couldn't comment about the proposal, and the whole family were debating and arguing constantly all night. They couldn't understand our old tradition, that many Turkish and Middle Eastern women don't like to marry after the death of their husbands, and they dedicate their lives to their kids and grandkids afterwards."

I sympathised with Mrs Muradi and suggested she could talk to her daughters and explain her point of view. I offered her family counselling, and prescribed a few sleeping tablets until she sorted out her predicament peacefully.

* * * * *

The rest of the morning session went quickly, with the usual cases of sore throats, hernias, coughs, back pains, sick notes and alcohol problems. I drafted a few letters and e-mails, and looked at urgent test results until around midday.

Dr Newman knocked on my door, wanting to discuss an issue with one of her patients at the end of her session. An anxious young lady with a tiny verruca on her hand (small skin lesion) was not happy that Dr Newman had told her to buy a treatment over the counter from the pharmacy, as we have to follow the trust's guidelines.

The patient kept arguing, wanting either to have the medication free on the NHS, as she was a taxpayer, or a referral to specialist. Dr Newman explained that was not feasible, as the specialist would return the referral back, saying the case could be treated in primary care.

The patient was not happy, and said she was going to lodge a complaint, adding that despite Dr Newman taking her on as an additional patient on her list, she was not happy that the consultation room was dark.

This was because Dr Newman starting getting a migraine, which she took medication for, but she forgot to explain this reason for dimming the lights to the patient.

Dr Newman decided to let me know about this patient's complaint, as I usually handle complaints with the practice manager. Thankfully, there are not many of them, and usually no serious matters.

I sympathised with Dr Newman and promised to sort it out if it came to my attention. She smiled and returned to her dark room to finish her administrative paperwork.

A few minutes later, Alisha, our clinic's senior nurse, knocked on my door to tell me she'd just received a text from Julia, the locum nurse who was due to cover for Alisha while she was away for a week. Unfortunately, Julia had fallen ill and had been taken to hospital for surgery.

I thanked Alisha for letting me know, and told her to inform the practice manager to sort out a replacement urgently. Alisha tried to apologise about this short-notice cancellation, but we agreed it was an emergency, and we should thank Julia and wish her a speedy recovery. I wished Alisha a nice holiday and reassured her that Jane, the practice manager, would sort it out.

I was hoping for a brief break, but minutes later Jane came into the room, as if she had been waiting for her turn after everybody else had finished.

"Sorry to trouble you," she said, but I quickly interrupted her, as I thought she wanted to tell me about Alisha and her locum cover.

"I've been informed about Julia, the locum nurse, by Alisha just now."

Jane frowned and looked at me with a puzzled expression.

"What was that all about?" she asked. I told her about the whole saga, and she nodded, saying it would come to her attention soon, and she had to deal with it beside tons of other matters.

"Practice managers are under increasing pressure, like the rest of their teams, and the majority of teams working for the beloved NHS," she said.

Jane added that she needed to discuss a few issues, firstly about the newly appointed receptionist, Emily, who was doing a reasonable, but not impressive job in her first three months' probation period.

"She usually arrives at the clinic late, despite repeated requests to come in a few minutes early, but she mentioned that she takes many buses to get to the surgery. She promised to improve.

"Also, some patients commented on her very pronounced make-up, and the very inappropriate dress for a surgery.

"You were not at our last partner meeting, as you were attending a trust meeting, so we were awaiting your opinion."

I replied that I supported whatever action Jane decided to take, as long as she followed the advice of human resources.

"I understand the issue of inappropriate dress, and we may introduce a uniform for the staff," I added.

I'd noticed that some of the young generation had different work ethics, but I recalled that in my childhood our parents taught us to dress properly for all occasions, and to go early to catch a train.

With a smile, I asked Jane, "What's the second issue then?"

"Well, the roof of the branch surgery was leaking, so we got a few quotes. But they were very dear. However, one quote was much lower, with a promise to do the work to a very high standard. He called himself John, the Polish builder."

Funnily enough, I'd just returned from a short visit to Warsaw, and saw their marvellous buildings and architecture, so I told Jane, "We are in a time of austerity, so I would agree with your decision for the lower quote."

Jane paused for a second, then said, "And another thing ... we have a new patient called Junior Davies, who just registered with us about two weeks ago. He had his first appointment with Alisha, our nurse, for his new patient health check. He has a history of schizophrenia, and is on no medications."

Jane told me how this patient had gone to Manchester to ask his cousin, who worked in the building industry, to find him a suitable job.

Junior's dad had given him some money and Junior was planning to stay there for a few weeks. His cousin welcomed him, they had a meal, a few drinks and kept smoking marijuana.

Unfortunately, they started arguing about family and religious matters, and eventually Junior left the cousin's house in anger, shouting that he was going back to London and would never contact his cousin again.

Junior took a few marijuana joints with him and kept walking and smoking the drug until traffic police stopped him on the motorway. They noticed he was drunk, and talking incoherently, as he wanted to keep walking to London, so they took him to hospital to be checked.

He had been admitted for a few days as he was feeling paranoid and delusional, and was aggressive with hospital staff. They started treating him, but unfortunately they had many emergencies and were short of beds, so they decided to send him to our local hospital mental health team in London, to continue his treatment locally.

When he was in a ward at our local hospital, he ordered a delivery of eleven large pizzas for the staff, and other patients, to celebrate his birthday. But the staff noticed his birthday had been five months earlier, according to his medical records.

The staff were also contacted by the hospital's main reception, telling them that a massive double-deck stereo system, with amplifiers, belong to Junior Davies, had been left by a delivery driver at reception, as the driver couldn't locate the mental health ward.

Junior had told the staff he needed to contact his family, so they allowed him to use the phone. That was how he'd managed to order the pizzas, and pay for the stereo system and a Bob Marley album, using his credit card, all to be delivered to the hospital.

The hi-fi shop hadn't realised he was a patient in the hospital, as he'd visited the shop in the high street a few weeks earlier, saying he would buy the massive stereo system when he had the money.

Even the main reception thought the delivery was for a staff member working in the mental health ward.

Staff there tried to contact Junior's father to ask him to collect the stereo system, as Junior was not allowed to have it on the ward, but the dad was not answering.

Jane continued, "So they rang us today for help, asking if we have any other contact numbers. We found his mother's phone number in the registration forms. We rang her, but she declined to help, as she was in Jamaica after having a big row with Junior's father, and now had nothing to do with both of them."

I told Jane to keep trying and send text messages. Hopefully Junior's father would eventually respond.

Later that day, a reception message informed me that they had finally tracked down Junior's dad, who promised to go to the hospital and move the stereo system and amplifiers to Junior's flat.

A week later, we heard that Junior had recovered. While the hospital asked us to continue his anti-psychotic medications and monitor him in the community, he had been discharged home to his flat, where we heard later that his neighbours were complaining of the loud reggae music of Bob Marley. Junior responded by using earphones, so he could continue to enjoy his music, and the issue had been sorted out.

Jane wasted no time in moving on to another item on her agenda.

She told me how a patient, Mrs Whitehead, had seen Dr Dikko, our dedicated, hardworking African colleague, who was the locum doctor for the day.

Despite cutting down on his work, with a view of retiring soon, he'd decided to take Mrs Whitehead on as an additional patient on his list that day.

However, when she saw him she said, "Oh, I was expecting to see the English doctor."

He politely replied, "The English doctor is not well today, but you can rebook the appointment if you wish."

But she decided to carry on, and asked him for her slimming capsules, as they had been stopped from her repeat prescription.

Dr Dikko explained the guidelines: we give slimming capsules for three months, and if they achieve a reduction in weight of about 5%, then we continue with them.

In Mrs Whitehead's case, capsules had been given for five months, with initial loss of weight of about 2%, but after that her weight went back to the initial figure.

Dr Dikko explored other options, like increasing physical activity, apart from walking the dog, and diet options.

He even gave her the option of buying the slimming capsules over the counter from any pharmacy, but she told him, "No, I want it on the free NHS."

Dr Dikko explained that we didn't give patients what they wanted, we gave them what they needed.

Mrs Whitehead wasn't happy and stormed back to reception, asking the receptionist, originally from the Far East, who was a new face to Mrs Whitehead, for an urgent appointment with Dr Newman.

She was told no appointment was available until the following week, so Mrs Whitehead stormed again, shouting, "Why don't you go back to your country! You're just a receptionist, I want to talk to the manager." Our receptionist calmly said she would ask the practice manager to contact Mrs Whitehead.

I agreed with Jane that some people didn't realise how much the ethnic staff contribute to our NHS. Frankly, without them the wonderful organisation would suffer a lot, and may even stop functioning.

Adding to our overwhelmed schedule, we now had to deal with Mrs Whitehead by phone calls, a letter or an interview, to make it clear that her response had been entirely inappropriate, and to draw the boundaries for any future relations with our staff.

I thought Jane had finally finished, but I was wrong.

With an apologetic smile, she said, "I'm really sorry, but this is the last request. An urgent safeguarding email has just arrived, and you are the safeguarding lead. Social Services wrote that they have visited Mr and Mrs Patel at home and reported what looked like a human bite on Mr Patel's right arm, which needs an urgent investigation."

I remembered this couple were relatively new to us. They had come from India to see their terminally ill only son, who had advanced colonic cancer, and to help their daughter-in-law, Manjit.

They stayed with Manjit for a while after the death of their beloved son. Manjit worked as a civil servant, and couldn't look after the couple, who were elderly and suffering many illnesses, so she had requested a social service assessment and help.

I'd visited them the previous week as Mr Patel had had a fall. A previous stroke in India had left him with a weak right side of his body, and he walked slowly with a walking aid. I noticed that Mrs Patel was struggling to care for him, and herself.

I thought to myself, had Mrs Patel been a bit angry and bitten her husband on his arm?" I didn't think so, as I remembered that due to her diabetes she had lost most of her teeth. So could Mr Patel have bitten himself? Again, I didn't think so, as his right arm was too weak to raise to his mouth.

I decided to call Manjit, who was on a lunch break at work and eating her sandwiches. I told her about the Social Services' observation of a bite mark on Mr Patel's arm. She reminded me that when I'd visited Mr Patel I'd requested a basic blood test, which the district nurse had done the previous Friday. She had trouble finding a good vein in his left arm, so she tried many times with his right arm, which caused a bruise that looked like a big bite.

That explained everything. Thank you, Manjit, and thank you, Jane!

* * * * *

I was glad that the staff issues were resolved relatively quickly, as I moved on to the routine work of checking test results and signing prescriptions.

There was a mishap with the prescription of one of our patients with severe anxiety, for which he was taking Diazepam – 5mg twice a day. He'd asked for his monthly prescription a week early, so I had to text him and brought it to the attention of the pharmacy that Diazepam would only be issued on the correct date, as it was a controlled drug.

I decided to grab the apple I'd brought from home as an emergency ration from my bag, and quickly eat it before I started the afternoon session.

I was hungry and glad to have the apple, as I remembered Alisha, our nurse, who used to work as a senior nurse in the local hospital, had mentioned that with the increasing work load in the hospital, some staff had no time to stop and have even a cup of tea, or an apple.

* * * * *

My first patient for the afternoon session was Mrs Dorothy Wright, a tall, elegant, smiley, confident lady, with plenty of life experience.

I vividly remembered her first appointment was at the end of a session, with little time to understand the physical and psychological aspects of a new patient so I could tailor their care. But in the first few minutes I realised we had many things in common. She told me she liked to read a lot, and she greatly admired the classic 1937 novel *The Citadel* by Dr A J Cronin, which was credited with laying the foundations for the introduction of the NHS in 1948. She even mentioned that she'd read it twice, a few years apart, just as I had.

Dorothy used to work for our beloved NHS as a medical secretary in a major hospital in the north of England. But she was made redundant, which triggered my curiosity to know more, as when I'd left hospital work I knew that the mounting pressure on the NHS meant it needed more staff, not scrapping an important position like her one.

Dorothy explained passionately her bitter disappointment at the state of the NHS, which in her opinion had been mismanaged in many ways. She told me that the hospital she used to work for had gone into debt by millions of pounds, so management decided to appoint a managerial consultancy firm to help.

They paid the firm more millions to advise them how to get out of this debt, and the advice was to reduce staff numbers, especially medical secretaries.

Dorothy added, "So they started by making people redundant. We had five secretaries in our office for four consultants, where the extra secretary was appointed to help with the research of the professor, and to cover for the other four secretaries on their holidays, instead of getting a locum, who was very expensive, and not necessarily familiar with the work of the unit.

"Then the advisory firm reduced the workforce down to three secretaries serving the entire unit, and with the intolerable pressure, some secretaries went on sick leave, due to continuing stress. So the managers had to pay more locums to cover, and it was shambolic, with more debt.

"The advisers then suggested that the letters dictated by the doctors, to be typed up by the secretaries, could be allocated abroad in the Far East, which would be cheaper. Our managers agreed and did that, and it was a very disturbing move, as letters used to come back with many mistakes, like paediatric (children speciality) written as podiatric (foot speciality).

"They replaced the word Dosette box (a box for medications) with Dorset box (a county in England), and the word laboratory had changed to lavatory. The name of a patient was changed from Moussa to Noussa, while 'outpatient department' had changed to 'our patient department'.

"The word 'done' became 'dome', NAD (no abnormality detected) was changed to MAD, or sometimes to BAD, and the house number in a patient's address was written as 29, instead of 39, which caused a letter to go to the wrong address, with a break of confidentiality. The patient never received their letter, and lodged many complaints."

Dorothy said the amazing thing was that the advisers had the audacity to ask the managers to tell the doctors to read and correct the letters themselves, something the doctors emphatically refused to do. So the other option was to commission the recently redundant secretaries to correct the letters, and that was where Dorothy's role came in, and they paid a lot of money again.

Dorothy found that was a clear case of mismanagement. She accepted the correction commission, which cost the hospital a lot of money, and it made her well-off enough to retire and move near her daughter, in the vicinity of our surgery, and to do a lot of charity work. She also had time to write a book about her mother's struggle in life during and after World War Two, and published it.

So, down to business. Dorothy had been suffering a very painful right elbow for a few days. I examined her and diagnosed it as 'tennis elbow'. She smiled and replied, "But I don't play tennis!"

"Yes, but probably you were using your elbow repeatedly," I explained.

"I was painting my bedroom last week and gardening."

I gave her treatment and an exercise leaflet to do at home. With a smile, she left the room.

* * * * *

Between patients, our senior administrator, Veronica, came to say that the local hospital laboratory had phoned, saying they were installing a new software and noticed that some women's results of cervical smear tests had gone into 13 men's records by mistake.

They were going to correct that, but they wanted us to delete the results in the men's records manually, adding to my workload. Thankfully, when I was going through them, the name of one, a Mr Self, who liked to complain, was among them. So I probably stopped him from having the opportunity.

My next patient was Mr James Duffy. The name rang a bell, and I recalled visiting Jim, as he preferred to be called, at home in the past, as he had severe back pain and couldn't walk to the surgery.

Jim had a fall a long time ago, when he used to work as scaffolder, and since then he had suffered back pain every few months.

His flat was a short walk from the surgery, which had given me some exercise between sessions. I recalled that he struggled to open the door and was accompanied by his over-friendly dog, which welcomed me by hugging my legs.

The dog's odour filled the unaired, smoky flat. It was very untidy, with empty beer cans strewn around the floor, a few crumpled cigarette packets, and three dirty dishes scattered on a filthy carpet.

At the surgery this day, he was dressed in an old black leather jacket and bright red T-shirt, with a distinctive cannabis leaf symbol and a few words underneath it, which I couldn't quite make out.

Jim wanted to get more pain relief, renew his sick note to take to the Job Centre, and to report to me that he had been seen by the physiotherapy team, who taught him some exercises to do at home.

But he'd forgotten how to do them, so I decided to print an exercise leaflet from our computer educational pack. Unfortunately, the printer refused to print, with a red warning sign saying 'change the toner', so I run towards reception and got a new toner.

I fixed the printer and gave him the sick note and his medications. With a few minutes to spare, I decided to address his smoking and drinking habits, but the minute I touched on the subject, Jim went into defensive mode.

He said he would try to stop smoking – but not right now. He was surrounded by off-licences and three pubs near his house, so he "couldn't resist" visiting them when he was passing by.

However, the good news was that he'd had a chat with his sister, who was living at Margate in Kent, and planned to move near her, away from this busy and tempting area of London. Hopefully, not near any pubs or off-licences, I thought.

Despite us disagreeing about the smoking issue, the atmosphere in the consultation room was pleasant. I was watching Jim's animated hand movements but he seemed to think I was interested in his T-shirt slogan, so he decided to show me the wording: *Man created beer, God created weed. Who do you trust?*

I couldn't offer an answer, so he told me he had used both of them – beer and weed –and compared them to the pain relief we'd given him, to see which one best helped his back pain. However, unlike the comparative studies we do in medical research, he didn't tell me the results of his study.

He added that he'd got the T-shirt from Pattaya in Thailand last summer, and he tried to tell me more about the famous Walking Street red-light district there. But his consultation time was running out, and with no hint of approval from me, he decided to leave the topic to another consultation.

"Thank you, Doc. And bye for now," he said, as he left the room.

"Bye, Jim," I replied, and nodded, with a smile, that no answer had been reached to the burning question: is it the beer or the weed?

* * * * *

My next patient, Maureen, was middle-aged, well dressed in a long navy blue skirt, in harmony with a light blue blouse, with a tidy hair style and trendy glasses. She was a well-spoken, educated lady, working as a drama teacher at a local school.

She had come on behalf of her mother, Mrs Wilson. Maureen had the lasting power of attorney because her mother, aged in her 80s, had developed dementia, which was slowly getting worse.

I sympathise a lot with my dear patients, but particularly people who have developed dementia, like Mrs Wilson.

I feel very sorry for them, and helpless sometimes against this merciless disease, which turns some patients from a nice, quiet, well-mannered, well-spoken person, into an aggressive, repetitive, argumentative, forgetful and illogical person, who can be a danger to themselves, or sometimes even to others.

Maureen had decided to sell her mother's house, and move her into her own house on the other side of the same street. Mrs Wilson's address had been changed to Maureen's address to get hospital letters and other correspondences, but by doing so Maureen had received a letter for her mother from the health authority to change her GP, as the new address was in a different borough, with a different post code, which was outside our surgery's catchment area.

Maureen couldn't understand this, as she herself was registered as a patient at our surgery – and nobody had asked her to change her GP surgery.

I told her that new instructions came out every now and then, which was why Maureen, in the past, hadn't been asked to change her GP. I said I'd try to find out what had happened, and I reassured Maureen that her mum could remain registered at our surgery. I'd let the staff know about it by writing a note in the warning section of Mrs Wilson's medical record.

Maureen was happy with that, but she added, "I mentioned to Dr Newman few months ago that my mother had had no annual follow-up appointment for her dementia, and so far she's never received one." I promised Maureen I'd ask Dr Newman to send a reminder to the memory clinic, to arrange an appointment there for her mother.

Maureen continued, "And while I'm here, Mum takes paracetamol for her arthritis, and you used to give her the soluble one, as it was difficult for her to swallow the ordinary tablets. However, the duty doctors keep changing it from soluble to normal tablets."

With a cheeky smile, she told me her cousin was a doctor, and they grew up together. He told her many things about medicine and the NHS, and he'd explained to her that the duty doctors did the 'switch script', which was software suggesting cheaper version to save the Department of Health and the government a few pennies.

I wasn't rushing to replay, so she smiled and added, "I assume they need to save many pennies to spend pounds on unnecessary things sometimes, as they probably apply the rule of 'penny wise, pound foolish'."

Before I had the chance to try to defend the NHS policy, or change the subject, Maureen added, "Have they forgotten their mismanagement of the old scandal of the PFI (Private Finance Initiative), where they opened the door subtly to the private sector, borrowed a few billion pounds to pay the debt, with heavy interest of more than £50 billion over many coming years, which caused some hospitals to close, and others to sell their lands to property developers to pay the debt?

"Or do you remember the saga of the Tamiflu? You can type it in Google, and see how much taxpayers' money they wasted."

I nodded, trying to calm Maureen, and thankfully she noticed that I'd got the message, and hopefully one day I can convey it to the decision makers – if they are willing to listen.

I couldn't find any political or diplomatic answer to her questions, so I said, "I'll change the paracetamol tablets to soluble ones, and I will leave a warning in the note not to change the soluble tablets to the ordinary ones."

"Have a nice day, Maureen," I added.

Maureen left the room, and got me thinking. I respected her knowledge and her point of view about our beloved NHS, but was she frustrated with the system as a whole, and the direction in which our country was going? She worked as a teacher, and reported that many of them were frustrated with the system.

She had probably been venting her anger at the information given by her doctor cousin.

However, I had a great admiration for her dedication and caring towards her mother, which reminded me of a markedly contrasting situation a few years back.

One day a daughter of one of our dear patients came to see me, and was very upset, saying that her mother's dementia was driving her bananas. She needed counselling, as her mum kept repeating stories and asking questions all day long.

I had to tell her a brief story I'd heard long time ago about a mother and her daughter who were having a walk in the countryside. The mother, who suffered dementia, kept asking her daughter, "Is that a sheep or a dog in the field?' and the daughter answered, It's a sheep." But the mother kept repeating the question, and the daughter answered angrily, "I've told you many times, it's a sheep." The mother kept quiet for a while, then smiled, looked at her daughter, and said, "I remember when you were little, and I used to drive you to many interesting places, and you used to keep saying, 'Are we there yet?'. And it was my sheer pleasure, every time you said it, ten, twenty or thirty times, to smile at you and say, "Not yet!"

I never heard the daughter complain again about her mother after that story.

* * * * *

Between patients, Veronica, our senior administrator, who helps us to tackle the ever-increasing bureaucratic load in the NHS, came to see me about some form she needed to fill in.

This was a safeguarding form from the social services collecting information about Sharon, one of our patients in her late 30s.

I had seen one of her three kids a few weeks earlier with a minor ailment. She had two other children from different fathers, however the third child was by Michael, her recent partner. Michael was not one of our patients.

According to Sharon, Michael was violent, abusive, a heavy drinker and gambler. He worked part-time at a betting shop. He was not always at home, as he often went back to his mother's house, usually after a heated row and a session of domestic violence with Sharon.

Veronica did her best to complete the form, but stopped at a question which she needed help with: "Are there any measures to prevent the domestic issues from happening again?" This was a good question.

After reviewing the records, one could see it was repeated theme, in which Michael would leave Sharon after a row, disappear for a few weeks, then Sharon would contact him for a small issue about his son and would invite him over at the weekend to discuss it further.

She would take the children to her parents to look after them, while she was dealing with Michael. After a chat, and a few strong drinks, the conversation usually became heated, with much swearing and verbal abuse, followed by physical abuse from both sides, resulting in a few cuts and bruises. The winner of this session was the one who called the police first.

Police officers would attend and call for an ambulance, then the hospital would involve the social services, who in turn would send us forms to fill in.

I asked Veronica to contact Sharon and make an appointment to see our senior nurse for a follow-up, and any further help from our teams, or other community teams like counselling, which Sharon had had before.

Unfortunately, the cycle of fighting and abuse between Sharon and Michael would continue, seemingly never to end. Some people would say 'Love is blind', while others would say 'Love hurts' and life will go on.

* * * * *

My next patient was Mr J, a tall, young, muscular, blue-eyed man with very short blond hair. He entered my room slowly and sat in the chair, making little eye contact. The pungent smell of cigarette smoke on his clothes and alcohol on his breath told me he was still struggling with his demons.

Mr J was an ex-serviceman, who fought in Afghanistan. One day during his tour of duty, his patrol came under heavy attack from the Taliban and one of his close mates, Mr D, got a bullet in the middle of his back, causing him excruciating pain. Mr J and his colleagues managed to sedate him and evacuate him from the horrific scene.

Mr D was later dismissed from the Army on medical grounds, as he was paralysed from the waist down.

The incident left Mr J with anxiety and panic attacks, which caused him to be edgy and irritable. He shot dead an unarmed Afghan farmer who he thought was wearing a suicide belt.

Mr J said he remembered the farmer's face after he'd shot him, with his eyes wide open, looking at Mr J as if there was one question: 'Why did you kill me?'

That face and the questioning eyes stayed with Mr J and caused him insomnia. When he finally fell asleep near dawn, he got intense nightmares and flashbacks.

It affected his relationships with his family and caused separation and eventually divorce from his wife.

After he was dismissed from the Army, he had a room in shared accommodation near our surgery, but sadly his flat mate complained he was woken up in the middle of the night by Mr J screaming, 'No, I didn't mean it!' .

A charity organisation that helps ex-servicemen, with a supportive letter from our surgery, had found Mr J more suitable accommodation. However, he felt very lonely and isolated, as he had no close friends or family around him. He developed severe depression, was on anti-depressants and other sedating tablets, and he smoked and drank a lot.

He was here today as the duty doctor had reviewed his recent blood test, with many results showing as abnormal. I also had to review his medications for depression.

I explained the blood test, and how his heavy drinking was affecting his liver, with rising enzymes. I told him he needed to cut back on his drinking, and he agreed to be referred to the psychiatric service for counselling regarding his Post-Traumatic Stress Disorder (PTSD) and his flashbacks, with another referral to the drug centre for help and a follow-up.

We agreed that he would come in for a review every three to four weeks, which he did. I was happy that he was engaging with the drug centre, our nurses helped him to reduce his smoking and gave him nicotine gum and patches.

In no time, he was on the right track, making good progress with his self-esteem. He no longer smelled of cigarettes and booze.

He mentioned that he had started going to the local social club to watch football matches on TV there, as he didn't have sports channels at home. With a shy smile, he told me he'd met a nice lady at the club. He'd told her about his problems and she was very supportive.

I was glad to hear all this good news and wished him luck for the future.

* * * * *

"Hello, God's Way." I greeted my next patient by his nickname. He was tall, well-built, of African descendant, and in his 50s.

On my computer screen was written: 'For blood pressure, medications, and please check his address.'

I'd known God's Way for many years since he arrived in the UK as an asylum seeker. He had worked for a few years, then had chronic back pain and hypertension.

He used to come in for minor ailments, or a health check, with a scruffy appearance. But today he was a different man, wearing a flashy suit, an expensive watch, and carrying an impressive box of chocolates, with a wide smile.

I thought he might have won the Lottery, but he said that we had helped him a lot and he wanted to give me this big box of chocolates as a thank-you gift. With a smile, I explained that it was our duty to help our patients, but eventually I accepted the chocolates for the whole staff.

I checked his blood pressure and reviewed his medications, but when I asked him about his address, his smile widened and he said, "This what I want to explain, Doc. My actual address is my council flat near the centre of London, but my registered address with the surgery is my friend's house nearby, where I receive all the surgery and hospital correspondence, as it was my old address.

"I would like to explain more. I got the central London flat from the council and after few months some friends advised me to rent it out to tourists visiting London, with a very lucrative return, and I can rent a room in my previous house, which was taken by a friend of mine for little money. The difference is in my pocket … and it's all tax-free!"

I asked him, "Does the council know about this?"

He smiled and said, "No, they are too busy in their offices. Even if they send somebody for a check, we tell the friendly estate agents to make sure the tenants say they are friends of God's Way, and they have my mobile number to ring me any time. I just go there and say they are my friends and I don't charge them rent. Even in the end, if there's any punishment, it's a slap-on-the-wrist fine, which I can afford. I've made my money already, Doc."

For a second I thought 'Subletting is illegal!' but it's not the only illegal act in this country.

God's Way paused and added, "I have been with your surgery for years, since I came to England. Can I stay with the surgery please? Especially when just before the election the government announced that any patient can register anywhere."

I just looked at him, but made no comment.

God help us all.

* * * * *

After dealing with a few minor requests from staff, my last patient on my list for the day was Zahra Abbas, a widow in her 40s with a grown-up only son. She was requesting a personal supporting letter, so I assumed it would be a short consultation.

Before I called Zahra, I tried to recall her history, which was detailed in a recent counselling letter dealing with her panic attacks and anxiety.

She used to be a very successful administrator in a big import/export company in Iraq, with a very good salary and a company car with a driver. Happily married with one child, lived in a nice villa in the suburb of Basra city, unfortunately, the Gulf War in 2003 claimed her beloved husband.

It ruined her life, as well as many lives in her beloved city of Basra, in southern Iraq. This city has a long history, and was one of the ports that the fictional character Sinbad the Sailor journeyed from. Basra was also home of noted Arab poets, writers, literary and religious scholars, and was considered in the past by some as the Venice of the Middle East.

Zahra left around 2005, when she seized the opportunity of a job in a branch of the same company in Libya, North Africa, where she stayed for three years before deciding to come to England, hoping for a better life of her only son.

Her good command of English allowed her to work and settle quickly in south-east London, and she worked as a teaching assistant in a local primary school.

However, she was nearly crippled psychologically by the sad memories of the past, which left her with post-traumatic stress disorder, anxiety and sometimes panic attacks. She was improving with counselling, but sometimes her condition was aggravated by even a hint of her painful past.

I used to see her with a smile on her face, but this time there was just a nod, and she sat in the chair with clear sadness in her eyes, which she tried to hide by avoiding eye contact.

I gave Zahra some time to gather her composure, and to ask about the supporting letter. She started telling me she had disturbing news from Iraq about her only sibling, an older brother, whom she loved dearly.

He used to work as a professor of literature and was multilingual, visiting many countries and representing Iraq abroad. He had decided to settle back in Iraq for the remaining years of his life.

But with increasing poverty and a very high crime rate, a gang armed with guns and knives had kidnapped his only daughter while he was at work, and in front of his wife. The gang demanded a huge ransom with a deadline for payment, so he sold his villa quickly, very cheaply, to a colleague. He collected the money, changed it to dollars, as instructed by the gang, and paid the ransom.

"My brother and his wife then went to collect their daughter at the allocated place in the main cemetery of the city, only to find her dead," Zahra told me.

The grief-stricken wife died a few days later from a massive heart attack, while Zahra's brother, despite taking multiple medications for high blood pressure, suffered a stroke later on.

He retired from work and became homeless, having sold his villa, although a distant relative offered him a sofa to sleep on and a hot meal sometimes.

"I need to help him, but I can't go there as it is not safe at all. In the meantime I need to bring him here to be looked after by me, so I need your help with a letter to the British Embassy in Iraq to facilitate his visa," Zahra told me.

"I don't want him to stay in what they call 'liberated Iraq' any more, and we shall meet with whoever invited these disasters to Iraq in the day of judgement for their handiwork of destruction, killing, anarchy, poverty and hunger, which are the worst weapons of mass destruction, started by the sanctions many years before the stupid war."

Zahra kept crying and I passed her a box of tissues and expressed my sympathy. I thought I'll write the letter while she was with me, but the computer screen froze and then cut out. I had to log in again with passwords, but unfortunately one of the passwords had expired, so I had to create another one. In the end, I decided to draft the letter at the end of the session.

I promised Zahra a very detailed supporting letter, which she could collect the following day, free of charge (letters like this would normally have a small administrative fee as it is considered private request, outside the NHS contract). I hoped it would at least help to alleviate some of the pain and misery the poor lady and her family had suffered.

She calmed down, and with a very faint smile, she nodded and said, "Thank you doctor."

"You are welcome, Zahra," I replied.

As Zahra left, I felt tense emotions. We doctors are human beings, at the end of the day, and many of us don't like injustice.

I decided to have a cup of tea, which I'd promised myself a while earlier, especially after such an emotionally-charged consultation.

While I was making my tea, a thought sprang to mind: 'At least count yourself lucky. You still have the autonomy to have a cup of tea'. This line had been said to me by a consultant friend at the local hospital, where he had the habit of having a cup of tea before he started his outpatient clinic. But a newly appointed young manager, who was a stickler for health and safety, asked my colleague not to take his cup of tea to his consultation room any longer.

Before I could move on to administrative papers and emails, reception rang to say that a Mr Everton was on the phone, sounding distressed about some inaccurate information in his medical record. He wanted to talk to the practice manager or me, but the manager had left for the day.

I decided to talk to Mr Everton, as I'd known him for years, and had tried to help him over his heavy drinking and smoking, drug misuse, domestic violence, and emotionally unstable personality. He got very upset when his beloved Everton football team was underperforming.

"Hello, Mr Everton, how can I help?"

"Doc, I went to the drug rehabilitation, as you advised me, but some of the staff were judgmental and made me feel uncomfortable. But they decided to help me, and they said that you wrote that I used heroin, while I don't."

For a second, I asked myself: how did I get that wrong?

But Mr Everton continued, "But that was in the past, Doc. Now I use cocaine."

Then I remembered that I'd written 'drug abuse', but I had been distracted for a second, and wrote 'heroin' instead of 'cocaine', probably as heroin was in his past record from the previous surgery. I thought, 'well both are the same family of opioids, both release dopamine (brain chemical transmitters for happiness), both are illegal, both can be dangerous and fatal sometimes'.

While I was altering the record and outlining the rationale behind the change, Mr Everton carried on explaining the major difference between cocaine and heroin, and was generous enough to expand the horizon of my knowledge about other street drugs, such as cannabis, ecstasy, magic mushrooms, LSD, speed, meow-meow (methadone) and the rest of them.

I told Mr Everton, "That's all fine now. The change in your record has been done, from heroin to cocaine." He was elated, and for me it was another happy customer.

I thought for a while that I could now close a gap in my understanding of street drugs for my coming appraisal (a compulsory annual check on what we are doing, and on our continuous learning and development), to show our NHS that we are up to date with our knowledge.

* * * * *

So, having my cup of tea, I started checking my emails about legal drugs which had been withdrawn from the market for safety reasons; other medications which were not available until next year as they were not in stock; invitations for educational meetings; new NICE guidelines (National Institute for Health and Care Excellence).

Then I noticed a new BAD guideline had just come out. I thought, 'If it is bad, why don't they improve it and have a good one?' However, it turned out that BAD meant 'British Association of Dermatologists'.

Going through the post one by one, there were letters from the local hospital adding to the mounting pressure on our admin team. Some letters, dated two or three months earlier, were causing a problem as patients had been told by the hospital to take certain medications, or follow certain instructions, but our surgery didn't have a letter to support that. Thankfully, the letters to the patients had arrived before ours, and the patients were kind enough to bring it to our attention.

Another letter was addressed to 'Dr List Pooled'. We didn't have a Dr Pooled, so as I was enjoying my cup of tea and had a minute to spare, I looked up the word 'pooled' in the dictionary and found that "a pooled means a weighted mean of means; you calculate a pooled mean by adding up the mean lines the sample size of each sample, and dividing this number by the sum of the sample size". I decided: No, thank-you, let's stick to other doctor's names that they write, like Dr Unknown GP, Dr Locum GP or Dr No GP.

The next letter was a hand-written note informing us that Duncan, a nine year old boy with learning difficulties, had eventually been accepted by the special needs school. His mother had written to thank us for our efforts. How nice of her to write, and it meant a lot to the doctors and staff.

Another hand-written letter was from Aysha, which put a wide smile on my face. I remembered her as a little girl, but she wasn't small anymore and was applying for medical school, one of the top in the country, and wanted some forms filled in.

I recalled her coming with her mum when she was five years old, and I asked her, "Hi, how old are you? And what do you want to be when you grow up?"

She answered emphatically, "I'm five years and eight months, and I want to be a doctor like you."

How times flies, and despite making me feel older, it felt like a positive energy had surged through my body. Filling out her forms, I was full of hope for the future, and for better things to come.

I decided to leave the rest of the paperwork until the following day. I collected my bag and made my way out, passing reception like a rocket. With a smile, and a 'See you tomorrow', I prayed there would be no 'Oh, Doc, before you go ...'

Out in the fresh air, racing towards my car, I spotted one of my patients walking around the vehicle. She smiled when she saw me.

"Hello, Olo," I said. Olo was the abbreviation of her name Olodumare, which meant God in her African language.

She wasted no time in replying, "I have been waiting for you, as I know this is your usual time to leave. Don't forget that I live in that street where I can see your car from my window. I couldn't get an appointment with you, and I don't want to see other doctors who are not familiar with my conditions."

I found myself under siege, with no escape, so I tried to give a polite answer, with a cautious smile, and said, "Olo, I'm sorry, but I don't do business in the car park."

She smiled and took a bundle of forms from her handbag.

"I need these forms for work and to apply for early retirement on health grounds."

I asked her to leave them at reception and added, "I'll ask them tomorrow to book you a double appointment with me in the near future. Can I go now?"

"Yes, thank you, Doc," she replied. I jumped into my car before she could utter the usual sentence from some patients: "There's just one other thing, doctor ..."

I switch on the engine, and peered at a warning light on the dashboard saying 'Engine coolant is low'. The same message had first appeared six months earlier, and it occasionally flashed on every few weeks. My trusty car mechanic had checked the coolant during a recent service and concluded that it was probably a computer glitch.

"Computer again. Drive, drive away," I said, as I pulled out of the surgery car park.

Driving home in busy traffic, I reflected on my hectic day, and as I like to learn something every day, I realised that I was getting older, my eyesight was getting weaker, but I was glad that my vision in life was getting stronger.

I had a feeling of relief mixed with satisfaction that I was still privileged to see different people, of various races, with or without a religion, and I was able to give something to other people. No wonder giving is one of the best things to make people happy.

For the rest of the short journey home, I had this thought in my mind: "Let us go home, have a few hours rest, and come back tomorrow for another lesson in the university of life, or as some people may say, for another day in paradise."

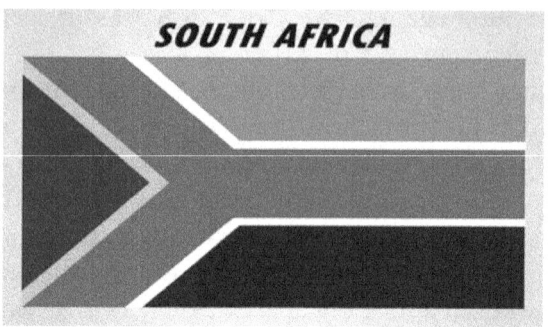

SOUTH AFRICA

Chapter Two
Joanna's ordeal

It was another very busy day in the clinic and I was glad when it came to an end, as I felt physically and mentally tired, and a little demotivated. This was mainly because of the increasing demands and expectations of some patients, and with endless documents, letters, and emails to go through every day, I feared we might miss something very important.

These days, doctors are under a lot of pressure, and some have burn-out, while many others are retiring early. With this burn-out, some doctors are just too exhausted and fed-up to really function properly any longer. Clinics are closing down all over the country.

Our beloved NHS is chronically ill, and instead of just covering up the holes on the leaking rusty bucket, we need to treat the causes of the rust in the first place. It might be a daunting mission, but it's the right way. The NHS is chronically mismanaged on multiple levels.

Offering money to help struggling clinics is a very good move, but it hardly deals with the cause of the problems.

I asked myself, 'Do we need help to cope with the increasing pressure?' and instead of putting that question to our managerial meeting, filling out forms, applying to our local health authority and waiting a long time, the answer came quickly to my mind: a quick-fix tool for coping is called music.

We know that research shows that music boosts happiness and reduces anxiety, so I clicked on YouTube and chose a mood-lifting song, and one of my favourites: *You Can Call Me Al* by Paul Simon.

I carried on working, and pushing my tired brain to make decisions on the letters I'd read, then came another fantastic song: *Gimme Hope, Joanna* by reggae singer/songwriter Eddy Grant.

I closed my tired eyes for a few seconds, and I felt like sailing away in a sea of memories, listening to the repeated name of Joanna, which stopped me thinking about work.

Coincidentally, a nice card from a woman called Joanna had arrived at the surgery earlier that day. She'd promised to send me a card with all her news.

I read it, while enjoying the rhythm of the song, and it took me back to events that had happened a few months earlier, when I first met Joanna.

Joanna had fallen ill after flying from England to visit her relatives in South Africa. She was covered by a travel insurance policy with an international firm I used to work for as a medical adviser.

She was admitted at a private hospital in Johannesburg, or Jo'burg as the locals call it, and the insurance company asked me to fly out to assess her.

The information I had about Joanna at that time was that she had repeated vomiting, abdominal and chest pains, a racing heart, and had lost her appetite. The medics at the private hospital had asked for many tests and were awaiting some results.

I made arrangements for the journey and arrived at Heathrow Airport for the 10-hour flight. Thankfully, I slept reasonably well in a reclining seat on the plane.

I was received in the arrivals hall at Johannesburg Airport by Bruce, the driver allocated to help me. He was tall, dark and muscular and in his late 40s. Driving a near-new black Mercedes, he had been working for the international insurance company for years, and had great knowledge about the city and its history.

He took me to my hotel, where I had a bath and something to eat and then went with him to the private hospital, not far from the hotel, to meet Joanna and the team treating her.

Dr Keogh, with nurse Van Graan, briefed me about Joanna's reasonably stable condition before we went together to see her. I introduced myself and we had short chat with the doctor and the nurse. I thanked them and stayed chatting with Joanne, to find out more about her symptoms of sweating, a pounding heart, poor appetite, feeling sick and apprehensive.

Joanna was an intelligent, very attractive young lady in her late 20s, with long golden hair with brown stripes, and big hazel-coloured eyes. However, her eyes gave the impression they were hiding some sadness. She was softly spoken, with fleeting smiles.

She told me later, that she worked as a supervisor for a well-known clothes retailer, where she met David, her partner. He was senior to her, and they went out for two years before he was promoted to a management role, and no longer worked on the shop floor.

Two weeks before flying to South Africa, Joanna told me she had severe period pains while she was at work. She felt dizzy with headache and asked her manager if she could go home to rest.

Arriving home, she thought that her younger sister Natalie, who was visiting for a few days after a row with her boyfriend, had gone out shopping, as she'd planned. Joanna noticed a few empty beer bottles and a bottle of wine, and thought that her partner David, who had the day off work, had probably invited a friend over. She assumed they had been drinking and then probably went out.

Joanna went straight to her bedroom, but could hear music. She opened the door and froze. She couldn't believe it: her partner David and her sister Natalie were in bed together.

She screamed at them and threw things at them while they were putting on their clothes. She chucked them out of the house and threw suitcases full of their belongings out of an upstairs window, with people in the street watching the drama unfold.

Joanna's family and extended family heard about what had happened, and Joanna had many phone calls from them, trying to calm her down and support her. One of her distant relatives, called Auntie Molly, in Johannesburg, heard the story and invited her there for a week away from London. Joanna accepted the kind offer, but said she didn't want to impose and would stay at a hotel in the city.

Her Auntie Molly was energetic, slim woman in her early 50s and her husband Nigel was in his late 50s, tall, dark and charismatic. They lived in a fabulous detached house with a swimming pool and impressive garden.

They invited Joanna over and treated her to a delicious meal and drinks on the terrace of the garden, served by a house assistant, who left after she'd finished her duties as she lived far away.

After dinner, Molly received a phone call with the bad news that her best friend had been involved in a car accident. She was in the operating theatre at the main hospital in the city of Pretoria.

Molly rushed off to see her friend, telling Nigel she would stay the night there and ring him next day. She told Joanna to feel at home and asked Nigel to drive her back to her hotel when she wanted.

Joanna and Nigel cleared the table and tidied the kitchen, then settled down for a relaxing chat about England and South Africa. They looked at a family photo album, with memories of the extended family. Joanna expressed her admiration for Nigel's achievements, as he was a prominent civil engineer, and Molly's role as a respected teacher. The couple had moved to South Africa years earlier and had done very well there.

Nigel and Joanna had some more drinks, then Nigel mentioned to Joanna how beautiful and attractive young lady she was, which she accepted as a complement with a smile. But when he kept repeating it, she felt uncomfortable. Nigel talked about his difficult life at work, and in general, then extended the chat to how the stress of work sometimes affected family life. Then, out of the blue, he hinted about sex-life difficulties after a lady's menopause.

Joanna read between the lines, and felt very uncomfortable about the conversation. She decided to have a cup of coffee and asked Nigel to order a taxi for her, as he was a bit drunk and not safe to drive.

She went to make coffee and Nigel offered to help. He came up behind her and held her around her waist, whispering in her ear that she was very attractive, and it would be nice if she stayed the night.

Before Joanna could tell him that was a very bad idea, he tried to kiss her. She pushed him away, grabbed her handbag and ran towards the front door, with him shouting at her to come back, as it was not safe to go out alone late at night.

In tears, she ran to a main road to try to find a taxi to flag down. Thankfully, she spotted a police car, which stopped. The officers noted she was a foreigner in some distress and drove her back to her hotel in the city.

In her hotel room, she sat in disbelief about what had just happened with Nigel, and it made her remember her distress back in London after finding David in bed with her sister. This flashback made her cry even more.

She suddenly felt very sick and vomited repeatedly. She also had chest pains and a racing heart, and was sweating. She called the hotel reception and a doctor was summoned.

The doctor examined her and decided to send her to the nearest private hospital, where the treating team investigated her heart and scheduled her for gastroscopy (camera to the stomach) to pinpoint the reason for her repeated vomiting, and why she had no appetite, just drinking fruit juice and water.

I spent a long time with Joanna, to establish a good rapport and try to understand the cause of her problems. At first she was hesitant and guarded, but she soon felt a bit more at ease when she realised I was on her side to help her go back to England.

It was clear to me that the psychological trauma she had suffered in a short period of time had caused her severe anxiety. It had made her frightened to be close to any man she didn't trust. She was desperate to return to England.

I gathered all the information I needed, reassured Joanna, and agreed that she could leave the hospital and go back to the hotel if she wants. I would keep an eye on her and facilitate her return to England as soon as possible. I asked her to contact friends back in England, to see if one of them could let her sleep on their sofa for a few days, away from her flat to avoid any painful flashbacks, until she saw her GP and attended counselling to help her through this painful ordeal.

I returned to the treating team and after a long discussion we concluded that Joanna's chest pains, sweating and palpitations were due to intense anxiety. Her blood tests and ECG results proved normal, and she had no family history of heart disease.

Her repeated vomiting was from the alcohol and coffee with the background of the severe anxiety. We added to her medications a little tablet – a beta blocker – to calm her heart and her anxiety, some milkshake to protect her stomach and some high-calorie nutritional support until she got her appetite back. Some light sedation in the evening would give her a good night's sleep.

Everybody was happy with this plan, and Joanna left the hospital and had a decent night's sleep back at her hotel. in The following morning, she had something to eat, with no vomiting.

She was happy to make phone calls to England to keep busy and to plan for a smooth return home. She told me she'd also had a very good chat with her senior managers, who agreed to transfer her to another branch of the company a few miles away, to avoid seeing her ex-partner when he visited the shop sporadically. Joanna also called her mother to say she was planning not to see her sister Natalie again.

We agreed to organise her return to England the following day, and everybody was happy with that. The insurance company in England organised everything, so I found myself with a day off to explore the city.

I rang Bruce the driver, who collected me from the hotel. He had a few ideas to show me many places, starting with a general tour around the 'City of Gold'. He mentioned the suburbs of Houghton, Westcliff and Parkwood, which was on a high hill overlooking the city, from where I could see the very affluent area populated by gold and diamond traders, with their massive detached villas with huge gardens, swimming pools, tennis courts, electric gates with very high walls topped with barbed wire, security cameras and uniformed guards with fierce Alsatian dogs. Some people called these villas "golden cages".

Then Bruce decided to show me somewhere completely different, and we headed south-west to Soweto, with its rich political history. In 1976 it was the centre of a student revolt against apartheid, called the Soweto Uprising, which spread to the rest of the country.

Soweto was home to the largest number of black people in city, with poor housing, overcrowding and poor infrastructure. Many shacks were made of corrugated iron sheets, but any visitor could sense the spirit of community, despite the obvious poverty.

Nowadays, according to Bruce, the government was planting trees, improving roads, creating parks, and boosting electricity supplies and water sanitation, while the town was attracting tourists.

Bruce drove me along the famous Vilakazi Street, the only street in the world where two Nobel Peace Prize laureates and anti-apartheid activists once lived. Today, former South African president Nelson Mandela's house is a museum, while Archbishop Desmond Tutu still maintains his residence.

We visited the Mandela Museum, enjoying the long history of Mandela's struggle before and after his 27 years of imprisonment, then we passed by the Regina Mundi

Church, which was famous for housing many anti-apartheid organisations and hosting many funerals for well-known political activists.

We drove through different areas, where it was clear the township had middle-class residents, with better roads and houses in a relatively affluent area, compared to the overcrowded original settlements of the immigrant mine workers in their matchbox houses of the past.

Bruce and I decided to have a light dinner and a few drinks in a pub, which was playing loud African music, with a mixed crowd of locals and tourists. It was a very pleasant time, with Bruce educating me about Soweto and its people.

After we finished the tour, he dropped me near my hotel on the periphery of the city centre, where I decided to walk and explore a little. I found a shopping mall and bought a scarf in exotic colours for my wife, and a fridge magnet to remind me of the place.

Walking back to my hotel, two young chaps were having a row with two others in the street. I didn't pay them much attention, but they got louder as I was passing them, and one of them pushed another one towards me. He stumbled straight into me, while the other one grabbed me, as if rescuing me from a fall, and said "Are you OK?" I answered, "Yes, thank you."

One of them hit another one on his shoulder, and they all ran after each other and disappeared.

I went to a shop to buy a fridge magnet, but as I went to pay I couldn't feel my wallet. For a second I thought I'd lost it in Bruce's car. Then I realised that the four young guys in the street were pickpockets, using a distraction technique to rob me.

I apologised to the shop owner, saying I'd lost my wallet, and he sympathised with me. I rushed back to the hotel and phoned my wife to put a stop on my credit cards and to ask the insurance company to send a guaranteed payment to the hotel, as I couldn't pay the bill.

I decided not to worry about this unfortunate incident, and aimed for a quite evening in preparation to the next day's long-haul flight.

I woke up early and requested a room service breakfast so I could phone Joanna to make sure everything was well with her. I was pleased to learn she'd had a good night's sleep and a small breakfast, with no more nausea or vomiting, and she was waiting eagerly to get back home. I rang the insurance company's head office, who were aware of my pickpocket incident and were pleased we are coming home.

I went down to reception to check out, and the staff knew about the pickpocket incident and had received the guaranteed payment fax from the insurance company.

They looked at me in sympathy with kind smiles, and I looked at them with the same feeling, as I couldn't leave them any tip.

Bruce was waiting for me outside, and we drove to Joanna's hotel, which wasn't far away. She was waiting in front of the hotel, with a big smile on her attractive face in the glorious sunlight.

At the airport business lounge, Joanna went off to visit the duty free shops and returned with a huge bag filled with chocolates, drink and perfume.

She told me she had received a call from her mother, saying that her estranged stepfather had been charged with sexually abusing Joanna and her sister Natalie. She had been waiting for this news for ages.

I was shocked to suddenly hear of yet another horrific incident involving Joanna, which would undoubtedly have contributed to her stress and anxiety.

Joanna told me it had taken a while for her to convince her mother about this terrible sexual abuse, but eventually her mother listened after her sister told her everything.

I felt happy for Joanna, and on the long flight home she was in a very positive and bouncy mood, saying the 10 hours had passed very quickly. At Heathrow's arrivals hall we were met by the insurance company's driver and Margaret, Joanna's mother, with flowers in her hands. She and Joanna hugged each other, with tears of happiness. Joanna introduced me to her mother, while the driver took the luggage and led the way to the car. Joanna agreed to stay with her mother until she sorted things out, so the driver drove them to the home in Lewisham, in south-east London, before taking me home.

During the journey, Joanna promised to send me a thank-you card after she had settled back in England, which she did.

As I read the card in my room at the surgery, I was very pleased to learn Joanna was happier in her work in the new shop, and the relationship with her mother had improved a lot. Joanna had also met a nice, honest man, as she described him. He had been at school with her and now worked as an accountant in the city.

A warm feeling flooded over me, when suddenly I was disturbed by the loud noise of a vacuum cleaner and doors banging. It was Maria de Silva, our surgery cleaner, subtly, telling me it was time to go home, for a few hours rest, and then back again for the privilege of seeing our patients and do what we can to help them with the pleasure of seeing their smile of satisfaction.

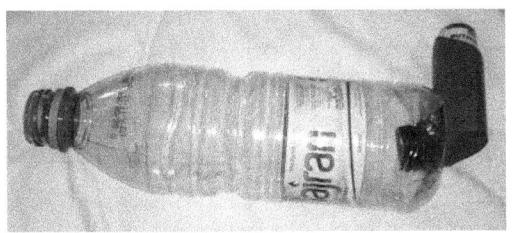

Chapter Three
Invention In A Bottle

One day I had an email inviting me to join a small group of medics on an educational visit to Kenya for a week. It was going to be a mixture of business and pleasure, and would be a good break for me too.

I consulted my colleagues at the surgery and my family, and both were happy for me to go. I answered the email the next day and was excited to be joining the adventure.

The group met at Heathrow Airport in front of the check-in desk and were welcomed by John, the team leader, who was a senior doctor himself.

After a long-haul flight of more than eight hours we'd arrived Nairobi, and were taken to our hotel, where we stayed for the first day, attending clinical educational sessions and some sessions about the local culture and history.

On the second day a member of our group, Dr Patel, a senior doctor in his late 60s, developed cough and fever. He was suffering from a severe chest infection. He was also diabetic and had high blood pressure.

John had let us know and had started him on oral antibiotics, which he carried with him in anticipation of any trouble. But Dr Patel's diabetes became erratic, due to the worsening chest infection. By evening he had developed an expiratory wheeze, even though he had never been asthmatic or a smoker.

John, I and another doctor from the group decided to visit Dr Patel, who was being looked after by his worried wife. We agreed that a Ventolin inhaler could help and we were lucky that John had one in his small first-aid bag. The inhaler helped a little, but Dr Patel found he couldn't co-ordinate the inhaler and his breathing, which made it much less effective.

He really needed something called a spacer. This is an empty plastic container, which is attached to the inhaler at one end and contains the drug from the inhaler. It allows the patient to inhale it more easily from the mouthpiece at the other end.

Nobody in the group had a spacer with them, and there was no access to any nearby open pharmacy at that late time of the night. A solution was needed quickly.

I looked around the room, thinking what we were going to do. Suddenly, I noticed a few empty plastic water bottles in a dustbin at the corner of the room. One, in particularly, was looking at me, probably asking, "What do you want from me?"

I looked at Dr Patel's wife and asked, "Does anybody have a pair of scissors?"

In no time at all, Mrs Patel disappeared and came back with a small pair of nail scissors, borrowed from the hotel reception. She passed them to me with a bewildered frown.

I picked up the empty bottle and fashioned a small hole in the bottom of it for the inhaler to fit. Then I sprayed the inhaler four times into the bottle and asked Dr Patel to inhale from the DIY (Do It Yourself) spacer. After a few minutes his condition improved dramatically and he used it repeatedly until he made a good recovery. We were pleased to continue our adventure with no more setbacks.

When we arrived back in the UK I immersed myself in my busy life. A few weeks later, while checking my post, I found a thank-you card from Dr Patel and his wife. They informed me he had mentioned the DIY spacer during his clinical meeting at work, which had made his colleagues smile. Additionally, a professor of medicine heard about the story, and commented that he used to do a charity work in remote places in a third world countries, and that DIY spacer idea could be very handy for poor people who can't afford the price of the spacer, or no availability in these remote areas.

That made me smile.

I agree entirely with the great Greek philosopher Plato that "necessity is the mother of invention".

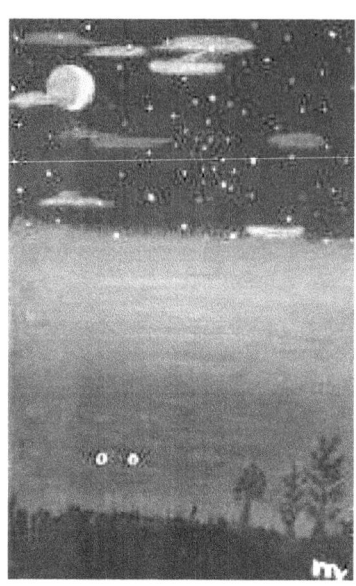

Chapter Four
The 7 to 11 Mysteries

I've known Steve Ashdown and his family – wife Julie and son John – for years. Steve, in his late 30s, tall, medium build, brownish hair and distinctive black and red glasses, was highly educated and eloquent, and was always smartly dressed in a white shirt and tie.

He used to work for the local authority, in the main council building, for about three years. He couldn't fully understand their way of managing taxpayers' money, and why the council had to spend all the money allocated to them, otherwise it had to go back to central government.

In my first encounter with him, he wanted a sick note for the stress he had from working with the 'bureaucratic machine', as he put it.

Steve eventually applied for a new job as an investigative journalist with a reputable national newspaper, where after two years he 'ran into trouble' by upsetting some top guns in higher authority. They didn't like what he discovered and wrote about. He'd made some enemies and lost a few friends, he was frustrated, disillusioned, and with the arrival of his son John, he decided to do freelance journalism for a local newspaper.

Steering well away from hot-to-handle political topics, he decided to write about food and drinks, and the best places to wine and dine in London, which made everybody 'content and satisfied'.

His wife Julie was a young, energetic lady, a bit shorter than Steve, with wide deep blue eyes, short blonde hair, and medium build. She had a 'go get it' attitude and was very healthy, with no past medical history, apart from the occasional migraine, which was severe and sometimes disturbed her work or social schedule.

Julie was a great support for Steve all the way and she showed her strength when she was working hard as assistant manager at a famous restaurant in London. She was pregnant with John and had a maternity scan, which found that John had a possibility of being a Down 's syndrome baby. A repeat scan confirmed this, and the couple came for a consultation with me.

It was a clear moral dilemma, in which some close relatives of the couple advised them to terminate the pregnancy, while others advised them to have the baby, and a third group were neutral, leaving the decision up to them. I sympathised with them and supported them as best I could.

Julie and Steve collected lots of information from whatever sources available and made up their minds in the end to have the baby, a decision they never regretted, despite many sleepless nights, changing nappies, frequent visits to hospitals and clinics, due to John's gut problems of diarrhoea and indigestion, hearing problems and many other challenges.

Time flew by, with their responsibilities and expenses on the rise, and luxury things pushed down on their priority list. Steve's journalistic output and Julie's hours were reduced, which affected the income. They decided to have a short holiday in Portugal and paid for it on a credit card – one of the few times they were in debt.

Struggling to pay their monthly bills and their mortgage, the financial strain affected both of them. Then came the Covid pandemic, and some terrible family news.

Steve's older brother Roy, who worked as an accountant in the city, was cycling to work when a foreign truck driver didn't see him in the blind spot in his mirror and collided with him, crushing Roy's leg and his bike. Surgeons at King's Hospital in London tried in vain to save Roy's leg. After the terrible accident, Roy started rehabilitation.

Steve also received disturbing news about his best friend, Darren, who had contracted Covid. As he was obese and asthmatic, he felt increasingly short of breath and his wife rang for an ambulance. He was taken to the hospital and put on a ventilator to help him to breathe, but his family couldn't visit him.

The pandemic affected many people, making some redundant and in deep financial trouble. This dilemma touched on Steve's family as Julie lost her job in the catering industry during the second lockdown, after the restaurant barely survived the first lockdown. The business struggled along until the second lockdown, when many staff were laid off.

Julie couldn't see her ailing mother Evelyn in her nursing home after she left her home, which had to be sold to cover the care costs. Julie had to sort out bills and deal with estate agents and solicitors over the house sale. Then the nursing home rang Julie one day to say her mother felt unwell and had to go to hospital, where she was later diagnosed with Covid pneumonia and sadly passed away.

Julie called the nursing home to tell them the sad news, and she asked how her mum had contracted the virus when she didn't go out or have visitors. The manager was honest enough, and later admitted that another resident in the care home had the virus while she was in hospital and had been discharged, as the hospital needed the bed.

Unfortunately, this information was only released later, when the care home GP received the discharge letter. Julie accepted her mother's fate but these events made everybody in the family suffer in silence. Julie, as strong as ever, organised the funeral and it was distressing to see only a limited number of family and friends there, due to Covid regulations.

All these events affected the family, but hit Steve more, as he used to suffer anxiety in his teenage years and while studying at university. He felt helpless, with a very low mood, and had no appetite for even his favourite food, and such poor concentration that he couldn't write more than a few sentences of an article for the local newspaper.

The editor was aware of Steve's circumstances but politely tried to encourage him to meet deadlines, but the pressure mounted on Steve and disturbed his already very poor sleep. At night he lay in bed, staring at the ceiling, and watching the green numbers on his alarm clock turning hour after hour until he finally managed to fall asleep around 4 am or 5 am. The following day he would be very tired, irritable, and quarrelled with Julie over trivial issues.

Julie noticed the changes in Steve and monitored him over many days, when his symptoms worsened. They decided to book a video consultation with me and to tell me about all the family's problems.

I listened to both of them, their voices reflecting the sad mood and the struggle they had. It was obvious that Steve was not himself, and was avoiding eye contact.

I explained my diagnosis of anxiety and depression for Steve, which came as no surprise to them, and I gave them options of treatment to choose. We all agreed to start medication, and I explained that as I liked to kill two birds with one stone, as there was a good tablet which could be taken to help with the depression and the sleeping at the same time. It should be taken around 7 pm, after the evening meal, and Steve should aim to be asleep around 10 or 11pm, to avoid a lightheaded feeling or drowsiness in the morning.

I outlined the rest of the common side effects and advised them to read the leaflet before starting the medication. I sent the prescription to their near pharmacy electronically, and I asked Steve to book another video consultation with me after two weeks to check on his progress.

Thankfully Steve booked the last video consultation on a Tuesday in mid-February, giving us a little more time if needed. Steve was sitting alone in his loft office, while Julie was playing with John in the garden.

I asked him, "How did you get on?"

"Well, where do I start?" he said, waving a few written pages. "I've written it up as a personal experience with the medication and I've sent a copy to you and to the newspaper. I'm sure the editor will like it, so do you, Doc?"

I replied, "Well, I glanced at it during my break, and I liked it."

Steve continued, "I started the medications and almost every night I had some strange little unusual event. When I read a new story book to John before he went to sleep, I was convinced that I knew this story already.

"On the second day, I was getting a fruit drink from the fridge when I saw the orange fruit yogurt tub for a few seconds with a red colour instead of orange.

"Another day after the evening meal we were watching TV when a car stopped near our house with music coming from it. I commented that it was very loud, while Julie said it was OK and not that loud. I felt I was probably imagining it and I didn't argue and let it go.

"On Saturday, Julie told me that we didn't do the shopping and ordering on line would take a week. We had run out of milk and bread, so I made a short trip driving to a local supermarket.

"While I was driving back home, the streets were quiet, with nearly no traffic, and I was listening to my favourite radio station while waiting for a traffic light to change to green. Suddenly I heard the radio DJ say, 'And very warm regards from Fay to Steve, I hope I'll see him soon'.

"I said to myself, 'If that is for me, then thank you, but there are thousands of people with the name Steve in the country'.

"I arrived home, hide the flowers and the valentine card for the next day, put the milk and bread in the kitchen and went to watch football on TV, while Julie was putting John to bed.

"The next day started with the romantic gesture of Julie bringing a breakfast tray to bed with a valentine card and small red flower in a thin vase. We had a toasted cheese sandwich, a cup of tea, and exchanged many nice romantic words. Then I gave her my card and the flowers.

"However, there were many events during the day which saddened the atmosphere a little bit. My best friend Darren's wife called to say the doctors would try to make him breathe by himself, without the ventilator, but she and their little daughter still couldn't visit him and were waiting patiently for any news.

"Despite this encouraging news, I became irritable and my mood was affected when I watched the TV news about Covid, with reports about the high infection rate, many people dying, and a new variant of the virus in many parts in the country. People were confused and more anxious.

"During the day I felt up tight, and I remembered the last conversation with my older brother, Roy, who had been affected by the lockdown. He used to go to a rehabilitation centre, seeing people who had similar disabilities, but now it was all video and telephone consultations. Roy was feeling down, and I felt frustrated not to be able to help him.

Julie and myself decided to be strong and positive. She was preparing the evening meal, with roses and candles on the table. She had bought John a red jumper. We had a delicious meal in a peaceful atmosphere, with a nice bottle of red wine.

"When Julie put John to bed, I kept watching TV and enjoying more wine. Strangely, the sentence 'Fay will visit Steve' came repeatedly in my mind, despite me pushing it away by concentrating on the TV programme. Julie came back, looking tired and slightly off colour. She kissed me and said she had a horrible migraine, and would take migraine tablets and lie down in the guest room in the dark.

"When she said the word 'tablet' I remembered to take my own tablet, as it was approaching 7 o'clock. Then I went to my office in the attic to get a cigarette box as I planned to smoke a cigarette or two in the garden, as I wasn't allowed to smoke in the house.

"Reaching for the cigarette box in the drawer, I saw a strange small rectangular golden paper box and I remembered that it might contain a small amount of weed left over after I gave up the drug.

"I rolled two joints, took some more wine, and went to the garden. I sat on a chair on the decking, near the outdoor gas heater, listening to music. It was one of my favourite songs of Otis Redding, (*Sittin' On*) *The Dock of the Bay*, which seemed to suit the circumstances we were going through.

"I was enjoying listening to the song, but oddly I felt it was the first time I'd ever heard it. I kept smoking and looking at the sky, with scattered clouds, which I imagined as waves of the sea coming towards me. I felt a strange emotion of positivity, then a sudden change in my mood, which I attributed to the effects of the alcohol and the weed, which I hadn't smoked for a while.

"I felt a gentle warmth running through my body, while simultaneously I felt as if the garden was shaking a little. Suddenly a shadow of a lady appeared in the middle of the garden, as if she had parachuted from the sky. Her face was bright but with blurred features, except for wide, glistening eyes. Her body was visible under thin, silky, transparent white layers of material.

"She said, 'Hi, Steve. I'm Fay, who sent you a message in the car that I'd visit you. This is a friendly visit to see how you are. You may say that I'm an alien, as you like to call us. Surprisingly, we consider you guys aliens as well'.

"I couldn't believe what was happening, but I asked her, 'Who are you, and what do you want?'

"She answered with a smile, 'My name is Fay, short for Fayrouz. I followed you and I've admired you for years since you were writing about corruption at the top, I was planning visit you but I had to wait till I reached 50 to be allowed to visit your planet. It's a similar age to the menopause in your universe, but without the hot flushes, as our planet is very cold. And on our planet we consider ladies of around 50 have reached maturity and they can visit any planet they want to. So I chose to visit you, but not, of course, to discuss Trump's impeachment or Brexit, but because I was very concerned about you and your family. I noticed your increasing anxiety and depression and when you wrote on your Facebook page, and I read it in the clouds, I saw the word DESPAIR, which I guessed was a reflection of your condition:

D: Darren's (best friend) Covid infection, and the Debt.

E: Evelyn, Julie's mother passed away.

S: Son John, and his challenges.

P: Pandemic problems.

A: Anxiety level very high.

I: Inhibition, and no desire to do things.

R: Roy, the brother, his accident and leg amputation.

'All these made you sad, and they made me very concerned about you, and that is why I have decided to pay you a visit'.

Steve continued, "It was true that I wrote the word DESPAIR on my Facebook page. I was puzzled about how she had guessed the acronym of Despair. I was intrigued to know more about her, so I asked her, 'Your nice name is a bit unusual for me', so Fay said 'My parents gave me this name because they were very fond of the angelical voice of the famous, iconic Lebanese singer called Fayrouz, who sings for peace, love and her beloved Lebanon. I know you Steve, you like to watch international TV stations like Al Jazeera English, RT (Russia Today) and

France 24, as the BBC is a bit economic nowadays on the international news. You may remember the recent massive explosion at Beirut port, on 4th August 2020, when President Macron of France visited Lebanon for support afterwards. He visited Fayrouz at her home in Beirut on September1st 2020, he had dinner with her and awarded her, the Legion of Honour, the highest honour in France and one of the most prestigious awards on the planet'.

"I was feeling cold and numb, but relaxed from the effects of the weed, and I asked her to come closer to the gas heater. She declined and said it was not cold at all, as on their planet it was always minus degrees. She added, 'Because you guys are interested in Mars nowadays, you know that the temperature in Mars averages -60 as Mars is many millions of miles away from the sun'.

Steve added, "I asked her, 'OK, I understand now your name. So, where are you coming from, and why you are visiting me?'

"She replied 'I'm from outer space, a different planet. I'm not allowed to say exactly which planet for 'national security', as you call it here on Earth, but I can tell you that you will know everything if you decide to come with me. I can tell you only about the place of my base, where I fly back to, and from there I can travel back to my planet'.

"I asked her, 'Where is you landing point then? Let me guess: it's the Nevada Desert in Arizona, or near Las Vegas, if you like gambling!'

"She replied, 'No, I descended to an island located west of the country you call it Norway, where the grave of the former King Herald Bluetooth of Norway lies, as we liked him on our planet, and as we believe in good communications between people on the same planet and on different planets, different races, different religions, and King Bluetooth was brilliant in that, and we were happy that you guys chose the name of a new technology of communications, Bluetooth, after him.

'We aliens, we like Norway a lot, you know that it is one of cleanest countries, with nature-loving people, it's advanced, with the highest standard of living, and it's one of the safest countries with the lowest crime rate in the whole universe. People there feel very safe, to the extent that many of them don't lock their bikes, they don't bolt their doors.

'They live longer than the average European, their health system is far better than many in Europe, including the UK. I know that one of your Prime Ministers once praised your NHS as 'the envy of the world', but he probably meant the Third World, if you asked your doctor, Dr Moss. Despite him being patriotic, a defender and lover of the NHS, he would tell you the truth, that he was so impressed when he visited a hospital in Bergen, in west Norway. He may also tell you that healthcare in the UK is ranked a lowly 18th in the world, and that a recent report mentioned the chronic mismanagement and under-investment in the NHS, alongside a shortage of staff.

'The NHS barely survives, only because of the hard-working, very dedicated staff, who are loyal to the organisation and their patients. The staff are really the heroes, and the angels of mercy.

'You asked me why I'm visiting you. It is Valentine's Day, the day of LOVE, the most powerful four letters in your language. Despite that, it is very underused or used in an artificial way, because many people are very busy with materialistic things in life, and some have even replaced this wonderful word with another four letters, equally powerful but for many different reasons: the word HATE, the word FEAR, the word WARS.

'Some people use these awful words to make money and profits. That is why you see some evil people throwing the seeds of hate between countries, tribes, religions and races to achieve what they are looking for, assisted by some politicians, a few religious preachers, and ideology adopted by some extremist groups.

'Every religion has many sects and branches, surprisingly every religion thinks it is the right one, and every sect looks at the other one being the wrong one. Eventually that produces man-made disasters called wars – another awful four letters that bring death, destruction, bloodshed, tears and misery to hundreds of thousands and even millions of innocent, peaceful human beings, who were living a normal live in the comfort of their own homes to find themselves the next day homeless in the street, losing almost everything, staying in makeshift camps in cold weather, forgotten by their fellow human beings, who called themselves rich, developed or even civilised countries.

'You remember the war they fought in a country with an ancient civilisation, called Iraq, with the excuse of finding what they alleged were "weapons of mass destruction". I wonder: are they still searching for them?

'I think some people on your planet had their moral compasses rusted, or one can say they are in bad need of calibration. The trouble is they don't see that, or they don't want to acknowledge it. Thankfully, on our planet we are born with a moral compass which works very well till the end of our life. So I never hide my admiration of the great people on your planet, like Dr Mahathir Mohamed and what he has done for Malaysia; the former Brazilian president Lula Da Silva and what he has done for Brazil, and when he said "Hunger is actually the worst weapon of mass destruction; it claims millions of victims each year".

He is a great man with great vision, and works hard against hunger and poverty. That is why all of us have to acknowledge his achievements, and those of great people like him.

'I came to you to express my platonic love to you and your wonderful family, and to highlight my concern about your fellow human beings on your planet Earth. You are a brilliant journalist, and even if you decide not to come with me, at least you know that you have a friend, never mind how far I am from you. I promise to support you and your family on your ragged path, to shed some light on corruption, which you have done before, or on the wrong things your fellow human beings are doing to nature and your planet. This mission is proving very difficult. I may remind you that your former Prime Minister, Mr Cameron, mentioned that word, corruption, in one of his last speeches and I think he was planning to work on it. But I never heard about that project again!

'We can't deny that your race has done brilliant things on Earth, like your industrial revolution, many inventions including computers, robots, artificial intelligence, mobile phones and many other good things. But as a journalist, you are aware of the many man-made disasters too, all over the universe, caused by some political clowns with their evil, short-sighted and sometimes brutal decisions, fighting each other in elections in the same country, or fighting each other between countries.

'You guys, on a personal level, are destroying the beautiful nature around you. You and your leaders are not taking global warming seriously enough, despite forest fires, floods, tsunamis, droughts, icebergs melting, sea levels and temperatures rising. People are still using cars, with more and more carbon dioxide pumped into the atmosphere. And diseases are on the increase: cancer, diabetes, asthma and hypertension.

'Look, we can keep talking about your miseries on Earth till tomorrow, but I know you have to go to bed around 11 to sleep. To avoid any hasty decision to come with me, I'll offer you 24 hours to think about it. If you type on your Facebook page, "Let us go", then you will find me waiting for you in the garden at the same time, to hug you tightly and fly towards Norway. From there we will go as one to my planet. I'll introduce you to everybody, you will live in my house and we will be very happy till the end of our lives'.

"I asked her, 'Why don't you tell me more of what I'm expecting on your planet if I decided to go with you?'

"She replied, 'Well, we are very peaceful people. Girls nearly all look like each other, and men too. We are all born with inherent gifts, like a moral compass. We all have the power to reach any distance on our planet, or even travel to other planets and come back. These powers you call super-powers or miracles on your planet. We have no religions like you, but we are aware that we had been created by an unimaginable almighty, who created you, us and everything around us.

'We follow our morals, so we don't lie, we don't steal. We don't have crimes like you and we don't build prisons to lock down people. Did I say lockdown? I'm sorry to use that word as I know it causes anxiety to many people on Earth. Hopefully your lockdown will be over soon and you guys can go back to your life, with business as usual. How much did you learn from this experience? Only time will tell.

'On our planet we have plenty of food and drink, enough for everyone. We don't waste food or dump crops to keep up the international price. We have no greed, no corruption, no cover-ups. We have no racism or any discrimination, as we are all equal – aliens, as you call us.

'We have real freedom of speech, and freedom to love, to marry or to stay single. We live anywhere we like, in houses, tents or caves. We can go anywhere we like on our planet and return to our base, as we have an inherent navigation system, like the sat-nav you have invented, or like the gift the pigeon has to return to its base. You may call it a built-in navigation system.

'We try to help each other and other people on different planets, which is why we visit you on Earth from time to time. I have never seen any visitors on our planet from your Earth, and to be honest it's better that way. People who are coming to our planet should be by invitation only, like what I'm doing with you. Otherwise, who knows, you may come to eradicate us from our planet, like what you did with the Native Americans and others. I have to admit I was surprised to know that after the American cowboys eradicated the native tribes, then Americans had the audacity to use the tribes' names of Cherokee and Apache on their cars and helicopters, like Cherokee 4x4 vehicles and Apache helicopters, to keep history in mind, I suppose'.

"I asked her, 'OK, Fay, I'd like to know: do you have anything to do with Julie's migraine?'

"She replied, 'No. I mentioned that we don't harm people or inflict any pain or misery whatsoever'.

"Then I asked, 'Suppose Julie didn't have the migraine and we were in the romantic atmosphere inside our warm house. What would be your reaction?'

"She replied, 'Good question. I would have reached you through many messages, like the one which came to you in the car. And I know you would have responded by coming to the garden for fresh air. Even if Julie followed you, she wouldn't be able to see me or to hear my voice talking to you, as I would convey my thoughts and words to your brain. Like what you call telepathy. I would only appear to Julie if she decided to come with you.

'One final thought before I leave you, as your 11pm bedtime is approaching. I know well that you are a good person and I wish you all the happiness, whether you choose to stay on Earth or to come with me, where I'm sure that all of us will be very happy. But if you decided to stay on Earth I'll try to help you to make your life easier and to feel happier. Good night, my dear friend. Sleep well, and happy dreams'."

It was the end of an amazing 7pm to 11pm conversation.

Steve continued, "The garden shook a little and a bright light appeared for a split second, then everything was back to normal."

Steve said he felt the cold of the night, so he switched off the gas heater and went inside the house, where things were very quiet. He headed to bed, had a very comfortable night, with lots of happy dreams, which was unusual, considering the weight of sad news he had in his subconscious mind.

The next morning, the day started as usual, with Julie preparing breakfast after her shower. Steve woke up very fresh, had a shower and went down to find Julie with a welcoming smile, as her migraine had gone. John looked well and was eating well.

Julie mentioned a phone call from Roy when Steve was in the shower. He was doing well with rehabilitation and promised once the lockdown finished he would come to play with John. That made Steve smile. He looked very relaxed and happy.

After a while, the solicitor who was sorting out Julie's mum phoned. After selling her mum's house, and paying capital gains tax, Julie was to inherit a six-figure sum, which made her jump for joy, as they would now be able to pay off their debts and their mortgage. They could afford a holiday abroad and put some money aside for John for the future.

At midday, Darren's wife rang to say that he had improved and was breathing naturally now, without the help of the ventilator. They had a brief video call on the mobile. Doctors reckoned that in a few days he would be discharged home to his family.

With encouraging news that the Covid infection rate was coming down and there was the possibility of lifting the lockdown soon, the rest of the day was very positive, with a relaxed and jolly atmosphere, until the evening meal and the medications afterwards.

Steve went to the kitchen cupboard and opened his medication box. He suddenly had the desire to read again the leaflet in the medication box before taking it. He read it thoroughly and smiled, putting the medication box back in the cupboard.

He told Julie he would not be taking the medication any longer, as he felt very well now and had an appointment with me, Dr Moss, tomorrow anyway.

Steve went to his office and wrote down his personal experience with the medication, emailed the article to the editor of the newspaper he worked for and another copy to our surgery. At bedtime, he hugged his wife and they slept happily together. It was a peaceful night without medication.

The next day Steve had an email from the editor, who was excited and agreed to publish the article.

When it was time for the video consultation with me, he went to his office and we connected.

I said, "Hi, Steve. I can see you. How are you?"

Steve replied with a smile, "Hello, Doc. I'm fine, and I wrote a three-page article. A copy had been sent to your email. I had to stop the medication as I felt well."

I noticed the improvement in Steve's mood and told him, "I can see that you made up your mind, and never wrote to Fay, because you are still here. And when you read the medicine's leaflet you realised what was going on, like the incident of the car radio message from Fay and the long conversation with her in the garden.

"I agree with you this is one of the side-effects of the medication, that in rare occasions it may cause hallucinations, which can be vivid sometimes.

"Let me add a few points to clarify: the 7 to 11 conversation was not the product of the side-effect of the medication alone, but because of the alcohol, the weed and the medication all together, it was a very extensive dialogue between you and Fay.

"All the information mentioned was stored inside your subconscious mind from your vast knowledge from reading, surfing the internet watching international TV channels.

"I'm glad that your stress caused by financial burden has been lifted, and your friend's health improvement is great news, along with good news about your brother and your son.

"I'll record the side-effects of the medication in your medical record, and thank you for telling me about your interesting experience. It shows that our reactions to the same medication can be very different.

"Good luck, Steve, and goodbye for now."

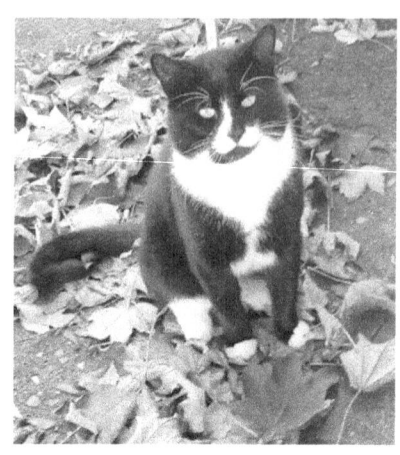

Chapter Five
From Tramp To Champ

One day we heard the loud siren of a fire engine pulling up at a terraced house about fifty yards from our clinic to tackle a fire that had broken out in the sitting room. After the fire, the occupant of the house moved away and it stayed derelict for a few months.

At our monthly staff meeting, Veronica, the senior admin, said she had noticed on multiple occasions a mouse running around the unused backyard of the clinic. She reckoned the mouse was hiding in piles of rubbish in the yards of neighbouring shops.

Veronica said she was scared of mice and asked for advice from the staff. Some colleagues started laughing, others suggested they could bring their cat and claim overtime for the additional work. Veronica replied that a cat could well be a solution, and with that we finished the meeting.

We never recorded this in the minutes, in case it was picked up by one of the many regulators of our services and we might be criticised for dealing with animals, as we were not a veterinary clinic.

A few days later, Veronica noticed there was a new visitor to the backyard – a black tomcat. He passed by near the edge of the yard, and Veronica decided to bring him some food to tempt him to stay around and frighten off the mouse.

She named him Frank –the first name that came to mind when she saw him. She explained to us later that she'd had a scruffy, academically low-achieving classmate in school called Frank. Veronica used to be kind to him, and now he is working as a top civil servant for the government (her friend – not the cat!).

Every time Veronica saw the cat, she tried to be kind to him and give him some food. She wanted to get close and stroke him, but Frank kept his distance and was reluctant to approach his food until she retreated back to the office. However, he began to trust Veronica and eventually let her stroke him, which put a smile on her face.

Soon she realised just how hungry he was – the fur behind his ears had changed to a brownish colour and started falling out, he looked thin and appeared a bit like an old tramp. On occasions Veronica used to call him when he was sitting on the fence at the back of the yard. He kept looking in all different directions until he located vaguely the source of her voice and spotted Veronica.

Veronica reckoned the faintness in his yellow eyes might be because he was malnourished, and that he was probably homeless. Frank was withdrawn and didn't pay any attention to any intruders passing by the yard, like squirrels or other cats. He tended to nap in a corner of the yard, waiting patiently for Veronica and other staff to come and feed him. The minute office lights were switched off and the curtains on the office door closed, he realised the staff had gone home and there was no more food and he disappeared, probably looking for any morsel of food elsewhere.

Days and weeks went by, and we found that Frank had now got a new nickname from the staff – Frankie.

After many sachets of cat food and treats from Veronica and her colleagues, Frankie started looking healthier, with the brown fur behind his ears turning black again. He trusted our girls in the administration office, and became friendly with them as he recognised their appearances and their voices. His eyes became wider and brighter, glistening, and he was putting on weight. Frankie looked muscular, heavier and healthier, and he was more alert when anyone called his name.

He would rush over for a play, petting and leg-rubbing, as if he was trying to tell the staff he had missed them, or that he was grateful for their kind gesture of bringing food and making his life easier, so he didn't have to chase the mice, which had vanished after he'd first appeared on the scene.

Frankie started to spend more time in the yard, and began to consider it as his own territory. He defended it fiercely against any other passing cats.

One day it was raining cats and dogs (so to speak) and Frankie was hiding under a small unused table at the side of the office door. The minute the door of the admin office was opened to give him some food, he rushed into the office with loud repeated meows, eyeballing Veronica as if he was complaining to her about the rain, or probably begging her to allow him to stay in the dry warm office.

Unfortunately his request was turned down as one of our staff, Shalima, who shared the office with Veronica, didn't feel comfortable when animals were around.

Despite this, her kind heart led her to buy him food, and even when she was the first person in the office she would throw it to him through an open window until the rest of the staff came to give him his breakfast.

A few days later, Veronica appeared at my open office door, during her lunch break, just after I'd finished the morning session. She looked excited, and with a broad smile, as if she'd discovered a solution to a big problem or she'd had a 'eureka' moment. She exclaimed with a hand gesture, "I think he's homeless!"

I thought for a second that she was talking about the new patient who had just been released from prison and had been discussing his case with me that morning. My confused brain wanted to jump to an answer, like applying to the council for some accommodation, with the usual steps of filling forms, supportive letters and then the waiting list. Thankfully I decided to ask her instead, "Who is *'he'*?"

I was relieved when she smiled and said, "Frankie, of course. He probably belonged to the tenant of the house down the road that caught fire."

Veronica added, "I had a chat with Jane the manager and we agreed to use some of the petty cash money to buy him a house to shelter in during rain, if that's OK with you?"

How could I argue with these two ladies, even with me being the boss? So I accepted their opinion with a resigned smile.

A few days later a big parcel arrived at the surgery with the name 'Frankie' on it. The staff opened it with curiosity to reveal Frankie's present. They took it to the yard, where Frankie was napping under a tree. He looked at them suspiciously and at the big, plastic, dark green-coloured house, as if he was asking, *'What is that?'*, and then he went back to sleep, as if it wasn't of any concern to him.

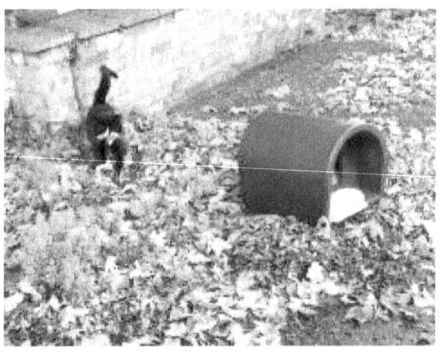

**Frankie looks suspiciously
at his new house**

Veronica noticed that Frankie more or less ignored the shelter. She tried to encourage him by putting some dry food by the entrance and by placing small towelling cushion inside. But Frankie would simply go inside the shelter, eat the food, keep licking his lips happily, and then hurry back to his usual place under the tree to sleep. Even when one of the staff tried to physically push him inside the house, he resisted with a big meow, as if he was objecting about the move. Maybe he reckoned the shelter was a dog house, so it had nothing to do with him.

I heard all these stories, and as I'm a cat lover myself, I tried to explain to our staff that there was a power struggle going on here. As far as I know, cats have a mind of their own, and Frankie had decided to be a free spirit. That was it and we had to respect his wishes. Thankfully the cat lovers in the clinic, including Veronica, agreed and accepted the temporary arrangement.

During the Covid pandemic, some patients were in high anxiety, and with the increasing demand and work-load on our staff, most of them felt really stressed. At these times they turned to Frankie as a de-stressor, and he was a real 'champ' at this job. Surprisingly it worked very well and they decided to give him an honorary part time job as the 'De-stressing Officer'.

I heard one day that a pleasant locum doctor was fuming, due to an argument with a patient who wanted many unnecessary medications to take with them while travelling to a European country, *'Just in case'* they developed diarrhoea, an infection of any sort, or muscle aches or headaches. All of these medications they could buy over the counter and we don't typically prescribe for *'just in case'*. Unfortunately, the patient threatened to lodge a complaint, which the doctor found unreasonable. So this doctor, between the sessions, decided to play with Frankie. Thankfully, after a while she was fine again and ready to deal with the afternoon session. Surprisingly enough, I heard her saying, "Dealing with animals is sometimes easier than dealing with some human beings!"

This was a sentence I'd heard before from a veterinary nurse patient of ours, and I think quite often it is sadly true.

Over time, the staff noticed that Frankie had at last decided to start using his shelter. Curiously, he always poked his head just outside the door of the shelter, as if he was thinking outside the box. From there he could see clearly in every direction the movement and approach of anybody. He soon settled in his relations with all the ladies of the clinic and with the cat owners and lovers, who would bring him some food to be added to his food bank. This was located on the unused desk in the corner of the administration office, with his name and a photo of him on it.

As time went on, I could see the spirit and the morale of the staff had been lifted. A new observation was that when the girls had their lunch break, they would bring a little treat to Frankie. In return he learned to play with them to keep them happy – certainly he was smart enough to realise there was no such thing as a free lunch.

Soon Frankie started to play his tricks on the staff – he never forgot that he was a cat. One day the girls in the admin office fed him his last meal for the day. The admin girls leave at 5pm, while our nurses work to 6pm. Frankie had jumped up onto the flat roof, which was just below the nurses' room window. He started to meow to our nurse, emotionally blackmailing her, as some people do. She was in the middle of catching up with her work before the end of the day. Our nurse Deborah rang me to say, "I may need your help."

Without hesitation, I answered, "Of course."

She said, "I think Frankie is either stuck on the roof and can't go down, or he's very hungry."

I replied, "I think neither, as I know the girls fed him before they went home, and he knows how to come down from the roof – I saw him sunbathing up there the other day. You can come downstairs and I'll show you."

I left my room to go to the admin office, opened the curtains and the door and called Frankie, who came running, jumping from the roof to another wall and rushing to come and rub against my legs. I gave him a little treat while Deborah stood and watched, open-mouthed and speechless at the cheeky fellow.

The next day we had a staff meeting, where at the end we usually discuss AOB (any other business). I found the staff discussing the petty cash money and Frankie's budget for food, and that made me smile. We were pleased that Frankie's budget debate was short and with swift unanimous agreement, not like other budget debates.

Time passed and Frankie decided to please his adopted mother Veronica. One day he was waiting by the back door, waiting for her to give him some food. The minute she opened the door, he rushed inside. I was in the corridor, going to the other offices, where I heard loud screams from Veronica and Shalima. I thought somebody had fainted, or something serious like that.

I rushed to their office to find them hugging each other and pointing at Frankie, who had a tiny mouse in his big mouth, with only its little tail and small head just about visible.

That explained why Veronica hadn't noticed the mouse initially, and Frankie was determined to enter the office to leave the rodent 'gift' under her desk – not knowing that Veronica dreaded mice and Shalima would jump in fear if Frankie entered the office.

I ushered Frankie out to the yard and told him never to enter the office again and to go and play with the little mouse at the far end of the yard. Thankfully, Frankie seemed to realise he was not welcome with his 'gifts' and went away, dragging his tail between his legs.

Many weeks later, we noticed a big, jet-black cat with an aggressive look was snatching Frankie's food and bullying him. She visited the yard almost every day and we could hear the arguments between them. We thought for a while that she was his partner and they'd agreed to live together in the yard, but Frankie was clearly not happy with her and her bullying attitude.

After a while, we noticed she had left him alone, as he wasn't interested in her, and Veronica helped by chasing the interloper out of the yard on many occasions. Frankie was getting thinner every day and Veronica voiced her concern that he needed to be checked, just in case he was ill or had parasites from the other cat.

Veronica contacted cat protection officers, who came to the surgery. They introduced themselves as Katherine and Katelyn, with their name badges written as Kat. I wondered: Did the cat protection organisation insist on staff names being shortened as Kat to fit in with the job?

They checked Frankie for a microchip that may identify his owner, but they couldn't find one. They wanted to take him away, and asked Veronica to put him in their cage, as he was less likely to resist her. Everybody could hear him cry after the cage door closed on him and he was going away.

A vet later checked Frankie, gave him all the vaccinations he needed, and decided to neuter him. The surgery was told Frankie would stay after the operation until the next day.

Surprisingly, just before we closed the surgery that same day, Veronica was told that Frankie was on his way to us. He'd had his operation and was recovering well, but they needed his bed, so they had to discharge him early.

Frankie came back with his discharge summary, which was type-written, unlike the hand-written, hard-to-read form from our local hospital given to our patients when they leave.

Our staff never expected Frankie's early discharge, saying the vet was behaving like a NHS hospital in discharging a patient early as they needed the bed.

Mona, our doctor in training, had missed all the stories about Frankie, as she had been away on a training course. Not knowing that Frankie had been castrated, she commented that it would have been a nice family for Frankie and his girlfriend, with little kittens that looked like him.

Shalima then told her Frankie couldn't have any kittens as he's had the big snip operation.

Mona replied, "Well, how about IVF (In Vitro Fertilisation)?".

Shalima laughed and dismissed the idea, as it wouldn't fit the NHS criteria. Anyway, she added, Frankie and his girlfriend were separated now, and Frankie was much better off without her.

Frankie started to gain weight again and looked happier without his girlfriend's nagging. She tried many times to creep up on him, but I think Frankie was more mature and wiser after his operation, and he kept well away from her.

Frankie also tried hard to enter our warm office, especially when it was cold or rainy outside, but all his attempts were unsuccessful. Later on we noticed he had gained access to a next-door neighbour, who welcomed him after their dog had passed away.

However, Frankie never forgot about us and used to come every now and then, sitting on the doorstep of the office and meowing. If the girls tried to give him food, as before, he just stared at them without touching the food, confirming that he was only there to say hello.

In the end, we had learned from Frankie how nice it is to live in peace and harmony, and to try to understand each another, while respecting each other's wishes.

At the end of the day, let us agree with our great learned colleague, Dr Sigmund Freud, when he said, "Time spent with cats is never wasted."

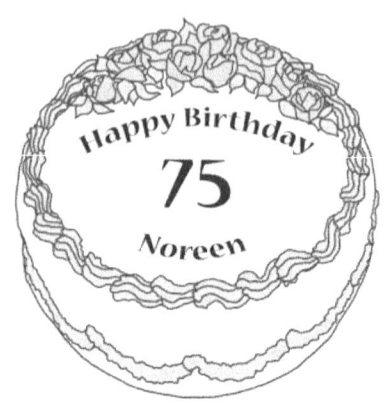

Chapter Six
Saving Our Precious NHS

The 5th of July 2023 became ingrained in my memory, as it was the day we celebrated the Diamond Jubilee of the NHS – the 75th anniversary of its foundation in 1948. The day began with grey skies and drizzling rain, but the sun soon came out to lift people's spirits across London.

I was watching the morning TV news while preparing my work bag with some patients' letters I had taken home to go through, as I'd had no time during the previous evening's session at the surgery before we closed.

The news was full of grim events, such as another fatal stabbing in London, a mass shooting in the US, riots in France and the continuing war in Ukraine. There was discussion about the ULEZ (Ultra Low Emission Zone) charge in London, and its effect on small businesses and on global warming. Thankfully, it was time for me to leave home before they could announce the Third World War, or an imminent nuclear Armageddon attack on the UK!

I walked towards my car parked in the driveway, when I spotted a light scratch on the front bumper, left by a red-coloured car. I thought, Could that be the car of the patient I refused to give antibiotics for his slight sore throat, caused by smoking and drinking? However, I was more concerned about a small but disgusting mess near the driver's door, left by a fox, I assumed.

Pulling out of the driveway, I almost hit a small dog that was off its lead. Luckily, the owner rushed over and pushed her wandering pet out of the way of my car, just in time.

I drove off and as I approached the mini roundabout at the top of the street, a long queue of impatient drivers were ignoring the right of way, with cars missing each other by just a few inches, and tailing each other very closely. Why the big rush? I wondered.

After I'd passed the roundabout, suddenly a door of a parked white car opened and thankfully I missed it by a few inches. Looking into the rear-view mirror, and mumbling a few choice words to the driver, I saw a petite blonde lady in a blue nursing uniform. I thought, 'She's a colleague then' and I forgave her, as she probably was thinking about being late for work or getting her kids to school on time.

Seconds later, an unmarked police car, travelling at high speed, appeared on the opposite side of the road, blue lights flashing and siren blaring. I was overtaking a cyclist at the time and had to pull back over to avoid the police vehicle.

All in all, it was just a typical scary drive to work in the heavy London traffic.

Arriving at the surgery, reception was busy. I spotted one patient, with an expressionless face, whom I'd refused to give Viagra at his last consultation. He didn't really need it and he didn't fit the criteria of Big Brother, I mean the Trust.

I said 'good morning' to the receptionist, Sandra, who replied, "Just to let you know that the phone has been playing up for the last hour, and the engineer is fixing it from the branch surgery."

In my room, I turned on the computer (thankfully I managed to log on swiftly) and looked at my patient list for the day. I recognised some names. I glanced at the accumulated prescriptions to be signed and the many test results, then checked my emails in case of any urgent matters. Thankfully, most of them were for promotional materials.

I went through the list of the patients with their different illnesses and complaints, tried hard to please everybody which is challenging sometimes. At the end of the day I managed to survive 'another day in paradise', as some people called it, despite the computer shutting down about 10 times, which really got on my nerves. I was glad to finish a few hours early that day as I'd promised to attend a small retirement party for John, my colleague, and a great friend. We had known each other for years, and we worked together in many hospitals during our long training.

John, who was tall and thin, used to call me 'Moss' or just 'M'. He was a dedicated, long-serving consultant in one of central London's most prestigious hospitals. Hard-working and down-to-earth, he was loved by his patients and his colleagues.

I drove to John's hospital, found a parking space with difficulty, and waited in a queue to pay the parking fee. An elderly man was struggling to pay with his mobile phone, and the machine didn't accept cash. He was being helped by the young fellow and his mother. New technology is supposed to make our lives easier, not miserable, I thought.

While I waited, I recalled a scene on the TV news a few days earlier of junior doctors on strike at the entrance of this same hospital. I sympathised with them after seeing one of their placards stating that their hourly pay rate was just £14 an hour. One of my patients had recently told me she wanted to change her cleaning job as it paid as little as £15 an hour. "Some supermarkets pay better rates," she said.

No wonder many young health professionals are struggling to get onto the property ladder, with many living in shared accommodations. One of the lady doctor's placards said, 'Even my mother didn't want me to be a doctor!' That made me sad, as I remembered that mothers used to be proud of their sons or daughters being a doctor.

I thought about other public sector workers, such as teachers. I have about a dozen teachers, teaching assistants and head teachers on my patient list, and almost all had reported poor pay and stressful working conditions. It took me back to remembering a top politician in the government one day saying, "Education, education, education." However, since he coined that famous phrase, standards in our health and education sectors have gone downhill, slowly but surely.

Entering the hospital, I went through the vast reception, crowded with people as it was visiting time, and made my way to the 5th floor, where John's invitation mentioned the staff room at the end of the ward, passing an assumed private side room.

As I'd worked in this hospital, I knew these rooms were designated for very important patients. Looking into one room, with to my trained clinical eyes, I spotted a lady who looked to be around 80 years old, frail and pale, with a slightly grey complexion. She seemed to have a chronic illness. Dressed in the hospital's white and dotted blue gown, she looked slightly distressed, either because of her illness or probably by the number of the visitors surrounding her bed.

Some of them were men wearing smart suits and ties of varying colours (mostly blue, some red and a few yellow or green), mingling with young ladies, who were probably their secretaries. Two tall gentlemen in dark blue suits were knocking on the door, talking with American accents. Their suits were marked with the pins of a well-known private medical company.

I glimpsed at a big cake at the end of the lady's bed, with Happy Birthday written on top, and red helium balloons shaped in the numbers of seven and five to make 75. So, I was five years out when I guessed her age at 80. I remembered the rule of 'never guess a lady's age', smiled and continued walking to the end of the corridor.

I entered the staff room to find the retirement party in full swing with light music, which John liked. I spotted him in his blue suit and wearing his usual thin gold frame glasses at the end of the room, surrounded by colleagues and friends, some of whom I knew.

I had worked with some of them, such as Sister Flannigan, who I heard later had quit nursing to join her husband's double glazing firm. Her pay was much better, with far less stress than hospital work, where some staff don't have lunch breaks, let alone a cup of tea, because of the sheer pressure of work.

I greeted Margaret, John's wife, who was looking well in a flowery dress. Margaret had retired two years earlier due to ill health, but had since recovered and looked like she was enjoying her retirement.

Suddenly, Margaret announced to everybody that she was going to play a two recorded messages from Alex and

Suzanne, their grown-up kids, who now lived in Australia and Canada. They wished their dad a very happy retirement.

Alex was a junior doctor, who went with his wife to Australia for better working conditions and lucrative salary, with a less demanding job, greater job satisfaction and more appreciation of his work. Above all, he was able to buy a house in no time, with the bonus of lots of sun, sea and fun.

I didn't blame him, and I remembered one day hearing a high-ranking politician commenting about young doctors going abroad and saying, "There's no need for young doctors to go to Australia." Was this politician living on a different planet?

Alex's sister Suzanne went to Alberta in Canada as a junior banker, and her fiancé was a Canadian gentleman. By all accounts, they were very happy there.

I grabbed a drink and a sandwich, and gave John his card, with a message of 'Happy Retirement' and 'Hoping to join you soon'. This was echoed by many of the staff in his ward.

We started chatting and I asked for his advice as I was also planning to retire soon. He revealed that he and Margaret had bought a retirement home in a quiet village near the Scottish border. They had been up there the previous week to order furniture and appliances and had a drink in the village pub, where the locals were very friendly. John told me the rhythm of life there was completely different from the very noisy London.

He winked at me and hinted, "There is another small-holding near ours, and when you visit us we can show it to you." In a further bid to tempt me, he added, "Who knows?"

John joked with a smile, "But we may need to cross the border to buy a cheaper fuel if Scotland decides to become independent. And if they re-join the EU then we can apply for dual nationalities!"

I was intrigued to ask John about the private patient I saw when I was walking in the corridor towards the staff room. John, with a grin on his face, replied, "It's a long story. I can't tell you here, but I promise to tell you everything when you come to visit us in the north."

There was something very unusual about John's grin, as if he'd discovered something really interesting about that mysterious lady. So I decided to ring my wife, and we agreed to visit John and Margaret at their retirement home the following week.

I couldn't wait for the new adventure in the north, and when the day arrived, we set off very early in the morning for the long drive, with many breaks and lunch. Arriving at their village home, I gave John a painting I had done especially for him, to remind him of London's landmarks. My wife gave Margaret some lovely flowers and chocolates.

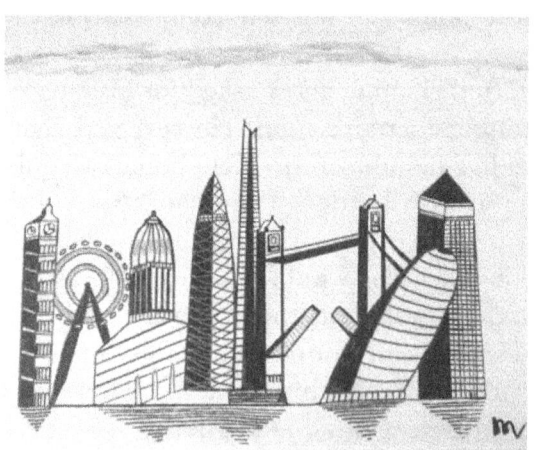

My picture for John of London landmarks

They ushered us inside the house, which was a massive barn conversion. We had a drink and went for a stroll around the village, where they pointed out the small-holding for sale, in case we'd like to join them up north when we are retired completely and decide to leave London for good.

During the evening meal, we reminisced about events from years earlier, when John had strong political views. He was president of a medical club and one day he received an unusual political invitation, along with others from London, to voice their opinions on how to help the struggling NHS. It was a good move by the government to listen to medical people on the ground, who understood the dilemmas of the overwhelmed hospitals.

John asked me to cover for him that morning, for about three to four hours, and he notified his team and the secretary. However, he declined to tell me where the meeting was being held and who was leading it.

I was surprised when he returned early and revealed that the "very important man" in 10 Downing Street had arrived late for the meeting. With an artificial smile, he apologised that he had to attend to an urgent matter and wished us good day.

"Of course, he had a photo taken with all of us for the archives," John said. "But at least I enjoyed the free hot pastries and tea. And as I'm a pet lover, I had a bonus that I met and stroked Larry, the "very important cat" of Downing Street."

I remembered that John, soon after that meeting, gave up any political involvement with these actors and stage-play politicians. He discovered that every time he tried to suggest a change for the better in the NHS, it was declined. He felt he was banging his head against a brick wall.

Margaret took my wife for a tour around the property, showing her their goat, chickens and two dogs. Back inside, they inspected the plants in the conservatory, and had a long chat about each one.

John and I continued our chat in the dining room, with John nursing a drink as he relaxed in a reclining chair. I raised the subject of the mysterious lady in the hospital room, who he'd promised to tell me about.

"Oh, yes", he said, "She's a very famous and popular businesswoman, with thousands of employees. When she was much younger she was the envy of many people all over the world, but she is ailing now, and struggling with chronic illness and poor nutrition. She is deteriorating slowly, and I doubt very much that if she continues like that she will ever make it to celebrate her centenary."

John told me her name was Noreen Helen Smith, and she told the staff she liked to be called by her full name. But they couldn't write that on the small identification board above her bed, so they just abbreviated her name to NHS.

"That's not to be confused with our dear old NHS," added John. "However, there are a lot of similarities between them. I've known both of them almost for the last 35 years, and both were celebrating their 75th birthdays last week, on the 5th of July. Both are deteriorating slowly, and if we keep ignoring them they will end in intensive care, with grave outcomes.

"Nobody would disagree with the long list of achievements and milestones of our NHS, over many decades, including mass vaccinations in 1958, the first British heart transplant in 1968, surviving the Covid pandemic, and still treating millions of patients, despite an underfunded, uncared for system."

John added, "Did you notice that Noreen's room was full of probably managers, but there was no named consultant to look after her, due to staff shortages? The NHS is very good at appointing managers from different backgrounds: from car factories, the banking sector, fast food and supermarket chains, from local councils, all in increasing numbers. They are appointed as ward managers, bed managers, cleaning managers, transport managers, catering managers, health and safety managers, and additional junior managers to support the senior managers. The end result, in some hospitals, is mismanagement due to some of them spending unwisely, with no accountability. This explains how the hospital budget is in the red, and the government will certainly need to bail them out at the end of the financial year."

John asked me, "You remember years ago you had an incident with the medical staffing in the Trust you were working for, where you agreed to cover for an absent colleague for a week during your holiday, and you offered to be paid just the ordinary rate? They advised you to instead use a locum agent, and you eventually agreed. You were shocked when you learned that the invoice from the locum agent was nearly double what you had offered the hospital. And later we realised that they did that for two reasons: to avoid all the administrative issues and to keep good relations with these locum agents. No wonder many hospitals go into the red.

"Do you also remember years ago there was an amusing report on the TV news about a very successful businessman being invited to visit one of the struggling hospitals, to tell them what was wrong, and to suggest a plan for correction? After a few days of inspection, observation and talking to each team in the hospital, he suggested many points for improvement, giving them a clear prescription for recovery. He pointed out clearly the 'cancer' that was affecting the hospital was due to mismanagement, and called for resources to be used more wisely, and better communications between teams, to avoid doubling the workload.

"He explained the theory of 'a leaking bucket with many holes', saying they needed to deal with the holes, not ignore them or to put plasters on some of them and keep pouring more water into the bucket.

"And have they implemented his recommendations for reform? I very much doubt it. It is a deep system of subtle incompetency, a closed club, cover-up culture. How dare any whistle-blower voice their concern! They will gang up on him or her, isolate them, and won't allow them back into the club.

"Ironically, they say that they apply democratic rules, following the path of their political masters in the government, where you can say what you like, but they do what they like. They believe in freedom of speech, but how dare you say the truth. The message back to you is 'Keep your mouth shut'.

"You told me about your colleague, a brilliant doctor who insisted on telling the truth and uncovering the dirt under the carpet. Eventually, they ganged up on him and sacked him. Thankfully, he went to another country and was more than happy there.

"Needless to say, the corruption in the NHS is subtle. Some people may argue that it is negligible too, but we can't deny that it is there, and it costs the poor NHS millions. Anybody can type 'NHS corruption' for an internet search, and they will see what are we talking about, not to mention the Tamiflu scandal to treat swine flu, with millions lost from the loose pockets of the government to the drug companies, or recently the many billions they wasted on substandard Covid PPE (Personal Protective Equipment).

"Meanwhile, we have many thousands homeless on London's streets, and for decades some of London's hospitals and schools still have asbestos in their buildings, causing cancer for young patients that we have seen during our careers.

"You also remember years ago that one of the top politicians said the NHS was the envy of the world. You have visited many hospitals in Norway, France and Germany, and you used to tell me about their cleanliness, their efficacy, their quietness, and their very high standards in every aspect.

"Meanwhile, we were working in a reputable London hospital, where we spotted some mice at the back of the hospital, near the mortuary. One member of the infection control team had the audacity to suggest having a cat to deter the mice, saying it would be cheaper than the expensive pest control consultants, as the hospital budget was already in the red!

"They are also pushing their agenda to promote the idea of privatisation of the NHS, which has already happened on a small scale, ignoring the fact that we used to have good service in the past with many public companies, like water, energy, the mail and the transport. Look what happened to them when they were privatised, with many subcontractors. Their main goal is big profits to satisfy their fat-cat top managers and their shareholders. I think a major shakeup and reforms are urgently needed. God help us."

John added softly, "I know I'm getting a bit drunk and saying a lot of reality, which you like, Dr Moss, and you write a lot about. So hopefully you will write about our discussions, hoping for a better future for generations to come."

It was getting very late, and Margaret and my wife appeared, announcing it was time to go to bed.

The following morning, over a full English breakfast, Margaret looked at John with a cheeky smile and said,

"Should I tell them about your first retirement project?" John nodded and with a grin started telling us about his idea. He had a blood pressure machine and thought he could use it to screen villagers at the Saturday market, with a little table and a chair, with some interactive chat about their health.

"It's better than consulting Dr Google, with no clear understanding, and I'd be helping the community, in case people don't go to their GP for any reason, like apprehension or no appointments available. If their blood pressure is high, I could usher them to their GP."

John had mentioned the idea to his new GP in the village, and he was delighted. He was very encouraging, and even suggested that John could join them in the clinic. But John declined, as that would make it like a formal job.

John looked at me and said, "I hope this idea won't come to the attention of NHS bosses, as they might send a panel to investigate what I'm doing, with lots of questions like: Do you have a licence from the council to set up in the market? Do you clean the blood pressure machine after every use? Do you calibrate the machine every now and then, like in the hospitals and clinics? Do you have a licence to practice? And if so, you need to have your annual appraisal. Do you give people medical advice? And if something goes wrong, did you mention it to your medical insurance to defend you? Do you keep a record of people you see and measure their blood pressure? If you are retired means you are out of practice, so do you need a refresher course to use the blood pressure machine?!!

"After all this nonsense bureaucracy, which we were fed up with in hospital and in your clinic, I would have to remind them that we used to encourage patients to buy a machine from the pharmacy and record their blood pressure readings. So do they need to answer all these same questions?

"When I mentioned my idea to a colleague in confidence, he suggested I could register that simple work as a charity, and Margaret could be the secretary. He said I could even franchise it all over the country, or even abroad in places like Africa. And I could ask for grants from the government and other charities, I could accept lots of donations, and with plenty of money I could take Margaret for business trips, flying business class and staying in five-star hotels. I could even apply for the prestigious Best Practice Annual Award.

"My answer to his suggestion was, 'No thank you. That's not me, and I wouldn't do that anyway'."

With wide smiles, my wife and I said goodbye to our great friends and headed back to London, where all these thoughts were crowded in my mind, and I promised to write about it.

My wife and I agreed that retirement is an end of a road which leads to another road. We should be enjoying this new road, with its adventures and excitement, doing everything we liked to do during our working journey but never had the time to do. Now is the time.

So long, my good friends.

THE END

The prequels

If you enjoyed this book, you may like to read the first three in the 'Drops of Reality' series. Available in paperback or Kindle on all Amazon stores.

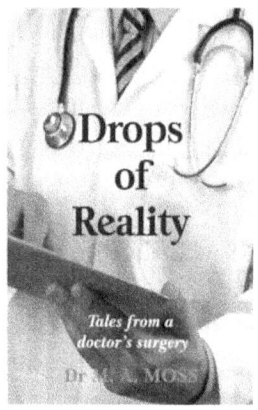

Drops Of Reality: Tales From A Doctor's Surgery

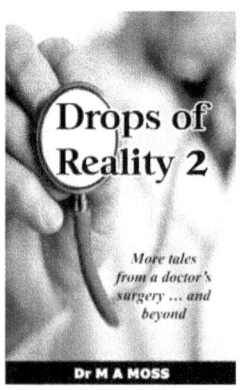

Drops Of Reality 2: More Tales From
A Doctor's Surgery … And Beyond

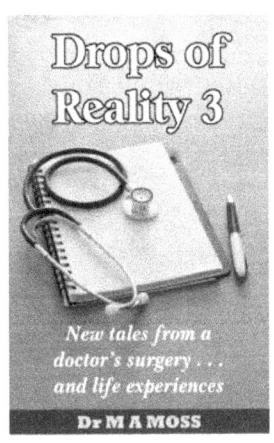

Drops Of Reality 3: New Tales From
A Doctor's Surgery ... And Life Experiences